THE ~~COMPLETE~~ PLETE
GUID~~E~~ ~~F~~OODS

In this essential guide, you can discover the amazing power of easy-to-find foods to help ease common conditions, including:

- acne
- muscle cramps
- osteoporosis
- backache
- skin cancer
- bruising
- headache
- sore throat
- dry skin
- flu
- hair loss
- nausea
- varicose veins

- toothache
- kidney stones
- migraine headache
- psoriasis
- sinus infection
- hepatitis
- anxiety
- bronchitis
- gas
- cataracts
- heartburn
- colic
- common cold

- ear infections
- diabetes
- gout
- anemia
- burns
- vertigo
- menopause
- premenstrual syndrome
- insect bites
- stomach cancer
- morning sickness
- laryngitis
- insomnia

and more . . .

Don't miss THE DOCTOR'S COMPLETE GUIDE TO HEALING HERBS, a Berkley paperback in bookstores everywhere.

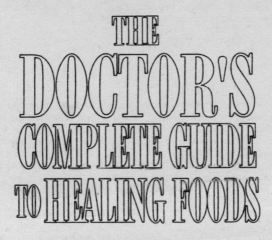

THE DOCTOR'S COMPLETE GUIDE TO HEALING FOODS

David Kessler, M.D.,
with Sheila Buff

**Produced by
The Philip Lief Group, Inc.**

BERKLEY BOOKS, NEW YORK

NOTE: Medical research about the healing properties of different foods is ongoing and subject to interpretation. Although every effort has been made to include the most up-to-date information in this book, there can be no guarantee that what we know about these foods will not change with time. The reader should bear in mind that this book should not be used for self-diagnosis or self-treatment; he or she should consult appropriate medical professionals regarding all medical problems and before undertaking any major dietary changes or taking any vitamin or dietary supplements.

THE DOCTOR'S COMPLETE GUIDE TO HEALING FOODS

A Berkley Book / published by arrangement with
The Philip Lief Group, Inc.

PRINTING HISTORY
Berkley edition / June 1996

ISBN: 0-425-15295-2

BERKLEY®
Berkley Books are published by The Berkley Publishing Group,
200 Madison Avenue, New York, New York 10016.
BERKLEY and the "B" design
are trademarks belonging to Berkley Publishing Corporation.

PRINTED IN THE UNITED STATES OF AMERICA

10 9 8 7 6 5 4 3 2 1

❖ Contents

CONTENTS

CONTENTS

Healing Foods 207

THE DOCTOR'S COMPLETE GUIDE TO HEALING FOODS

❖ Introduction

Food and Your Health

Everyone knows that eating right helps keep you healthy. But what exactly is eating right? Even more precisely, what does eating right mean for *you?* There's no simple answer to this essential question. A lot depends on your overall health and your age, to say nothing of your lifestyle and personal likes and dislikes. If you have a particular health problem, changing your diet or eating specific foods may help relieve symptoms or even play a role in curing the condition. In most cases, however, diet is only one aspect of the treatment. Before you make any major changes in your diet, whether to treat a health problem or for any other reason, discuss them with your doctor.

The Basics of a Healthy Diet

You can enjoy overall better health and reduce your risk of getting diseases, such as cancer and heart disease, by following the basic dietary guidelines developed by the United States Department of Agriculture and the Department of Health and Human Services. These are the best, most up-to-date, and most sensible guidelines now available. They're

1

based on serious science, not anecdotal evidence, and they work. There are seven simple, basic, logical guidelines:

Eat a variety of foods. Paradoxically, as researchers learn more and more about the health-giving properties of the foods we eat, they realize even more how complex those foods—and our responses to them—are. Because you need more than forty different nutrients for good health, no one food, food component, or food supplement is a magic bullet that can do it all. By eating a variety of foods over the course of a day, you get the energy, protein, vitamins, minerals, and fiber you need. You also keep yourself from getting bored by your food. It's much easier to stick to a healthy diet if it remains interesting and tasty.

Maintain a healthy weight. As a physician, I can't stress this enough. If you are overweight, you greatly increase your chances of diabetes, stroke, high blood pressure, heart disease, and certain cancers. Being overweight makes conditions such as arthritis worse. What is a healthy weight for you? There's no exact answer, only general guidelines. Happily, you don't have to look like a fashion model to be within the suggested weights for your height and age. In fact, recent research suggests that you can get a little heavier as you get older without added health risks, although exactly how much heavier is still unclear.

Choose a diet low in fat, saturated fat, and cholesterol. Fat contains over twice the calories of an equal amount of carbohydrates or protein. A low-fat diet reduces your risk of obesity, heart disease, and certain types of cancer. (The different types of fat and why you should limit them will be discussed below.)

Choose a diet with plenty of vegetables, fruits, and grains. These foods provide vitamins, minerals, fiber, and complex carbohydrates. They also contain numerous complex compounds called *phytochemicals* that can help your body fight off illness and keep you healthy. (See page 11 for a complete explanation.)

Use sugar only in moderation. A diet loaded with sugar has too many calories and too few nutrients. Sugar is consumed liberally in the American diet. It's used most commonly as white table sugar (sucrose), but molasses, brown sugar, raw sugar, glucose (dextrose), fructose, maltose, lactose, honey, syrup, corn syrup, high-fructose corn sweetener, and fruit juice concentrate are all sugars as well. They are all high in calories and low in nutrition—even the unrefined or "natural" sugars. In fact, honey has more calories than the same amount of table sugar. Read food labels carefully to find the hidden sugar in prepared foods, such as salad dressings, baked goods, breakfast cereals, and other foods. A food is likely to be high in sugar if its ingredient list shows any form of sugar as the first or second ingredient or if it lists several different sugars.

Use salt and sodium only in moderation. Table salt contains sodium and chloride, two minerals that are essential to your body. However, most Americans eat far too much salt and sodium, because these are frequently added to processed foods. Doctors agree that limiting the salt in your diet is desirable and can help prevent high blood pressure, although they disagree somewhat on how strict those limits should be. Some doctors feel that up to 3,000 milligrams a day is acceptable if you are in good health; others feel that 2,400 milligrams a day should be the maximum. (There are about 2,000 milligrams of salt in a teaspoon.) To cut back on salt, add table salt to your food sparingly or not at all. Try to avoid canned and processed foods, convenience foods, and salty condiments and snacks. Just two ounces of bologna contain 580 milligrams of salt.

If you drink alcoholic beverages, do so in moderation. Alcohol supplies calories but little or no nutrition. Alcohol is the cause of many health problems and can make other health problems worse. It is also the cause of many injuries from falls and accidents. Don't drink alcohol if:

- You are trying to conceive, are pregnant, or think you might be
- You plan to drive or engage in other activities that require attention and skill

- You are taking any sort of prescription or nonprescription drug
- You have trouble controlling how much you drink

Recent research shows that people who regularly have a drink or two a day over a period of years have lower rates of heart disease. If you don't already drink moderately on a regular basis, however, you are not likely to benefit from adding alcohol to your diet. Moderate drinking means no more than one drink a day for a woman and two drinks a day for a man. A drink is defined as 12 ounces of beer (one can), 5 ounces of wine, or 1 1/2 ounces (one shot) of distilled spirits (80 proof).

The Food Pyramid

The food pyramid offers general guidelines for a nutritious diet. The food pyramid concept replaces the familiar four food groups many of us grew up with, so it can take a little getting used to. The base of the food pyramid is grains: bread, cereal, rice, and pasta. The recommendation is for six to eleven servings of these foods a day. Next up on the pyramid are the fruit and vegetable groups. The recommended amount of vegetables is three to five servings daily; for fruits, which are high in natural sugars, the recommendation is two to four servings. Nearing the top of the pyramid are the dairy foods group and the group containing meat, poultry, fish, beans, eggs, and nuts. From the dairy food group, two to three servings daily are recommended. Two to three servings from the meat group are suggested as well. At the top of the pyramid are fats, oils, and sweets. Use these only sparingly.

Many people find the serving recommendations in the food pyramid confusing. It seems like a lot to eat, until you realize that each serving is actually quite small. For example, a slice of bread counts as one serving; a serving of natural cheese is just 1 1/2 ounces, and a serving of fresh tomatoes is just half a cup. So, if you have an apple and a low-fat cheese sandwich with tomatoes on whole wheat bread for lunch, you have had a healthy meal that contains two servings from the grain group and one each from the dairy, fruit, and vegetable groups. At that rate, it's easy to get your recommended servings every day. (See the chart on page 16 for more information.)

Some nutritionists and physicians feel that the food pyramid still places too much emphasis on dairy and meat products. Remember that these are guidelines, not rigid rules. It certainly wouldn't hurt most people to eat more grains, fruits, and vegetables and less meat and cheese than the pyramid suggests.

A Closer Look at Fat

The benefits of a low-fat diet are clear: reduced risk of obesity, heart disease, and some cancers. What's often unclear is exactly what a low-fat diet is. Most physicians and nutritionists agree that no more than 30 percent of your daily calories should come from fat. (Some would go a lot further and say that much less fat is better, but the evidence for this is somewhat contradictory.) In the average 2,200 calorie diet, then, about 660 calories should come from fat. Since approximately 9 calories are in each gram of fat, your diet would contain about 73 grams of fat. To get a better handle on this, figure that there are about 4 grams of fat in a teaspoon. (Imagine yourself swallowing 18 teaspoons of fat a day, and remember that the average American actually eats even more.)

The demonization of fat can be very confusing. First, bear in mind that your body needs fat. It is a rich source of energy. Gram for gram, fat gives you more than twice as much energy as an equivalent amount of protein. Your body also stores energy by converting excess protein and carbohydrate to body fat, and you need some stored fat for times when you can't eat enough or need extra energy. Fats are essential for making the membranes of your body's cells, for cushioning your internal organs and protecting them from injury, and for absorbing vitamins A, D, E, and K.

Fats are organic substances found in plant and animal foods. Fats are also called fatty acids because of their molecular structure. The structure of fat is quite complex, and how your body utilizes fat is even more complicated. To put it in simplified terms, fat is made up of hydrogen, carbon, and oxygen. A typical fat molecule consists of three fatty acids and one glycerol. The fatty acid parts of the molecule consist of chains of hydrogen and carbon atoms. The structure of the chains defines the type of fat. Almost all fats are a mixture of different types, with one type more prevalent.

Saturated fats. When all the carbon atoms in the fatty acid chains are linked to hydrogen atoms, the result is a saturated fat. Saturated fats such a lard or vegetable shortening are generally solid at room temperature. Saturated fats are found in the largest amounts in meat and dairy products and in some vegetable fats such as coconut oil, palm oil, and palm kernel oil, which are often called tropical oils. Eating too much saturated fat can raise your levels of blood cholesterol. To reduce your risk of heart disease, no more than 10 percent of your total daily calories or about a third of your daily fat intake should come from saturated fats. Saturated fats are often hidden in many foods. For example, nondairy creamers and commercial baked goods are often high in saturated fats. Read the ingredients list carefully.

Monounsaturated fats. If only some of the carbon atoms in the fatty acid chains are linked to hydrogen atoms, the remaining carbon atoms link up with other carbon atoms to form double bonds. A fat that has just one of these double carbon bonds is called a monounsaturated fat. Examples of monounsaturated fats include olive oil, peanut oil, and canola oil. For complex chemical reasons, monounsaturated fats can actually help reduce blood cholesterol levels. Try to make most of your fat intake be in the form of monounsaturated fat.

Polyunsaturated fats. If two or more of the carbon atoms in the fatty acid chains are double-bonded to other carbon atoms instead of hydrogen atoms, the fat is polyunsaturated. Examples of polyunsaturated fat include safflower oil, sunflower oil, corn oil, soybean oil, and cottonseed oil.

Essential fatty acids Your body converts some of the fat you eat into other types of fatty acids that are essential for normal functioning. These fatty acids are used to build your cell membranes and are the building blocks for vital hormonelike substances such as prostaglandins and thromboxane. Linoleic acid and linolenic acid, however, can't be made by your body. These must come from your diet. In general, you can get these polyunsaturated fatty acids by eating a normal diet. Linolenic acid, also known as omega-6 fatty acid, is found in all natural fats, especially vegetable oils. One form of omega-6 fatty acid, gamma linolenic oil (GLA), is found in evening primrose oil, borage seed oil, and black currant oil. Linoleic acid, also known as omega-3 fatty acid, is found in linseed (flaxseed) oil, but the most common dietary source is fish and fish oil. One form of linoleic acid found in fish oil, eicosapentanoic acid (EPA), is the type usually sold at health food stores in capsules.

Cholesterol. Fat and cholesterol are not the same thing. Cholesterol is a fatlike substance found in all animal foods, including meat, poultry, egg yolks, milk and dairy products, and fish. It's also produced by your liver. Plant foods usually contain some fat but never have any cholesterol. This is why manufacturers can claim that a food high in calories and saturated fat—a cookie made with palm oil, for example—has no cholesterol. They are attempting to fool unwary consumers into thinking that the food is somehow healthier.

Cholesterol and fat are carried to your cells by your bloodstream. But since fats can't dissolve in water (and blood is made up mostly of water), they have to be wrapped inside little packets of protein called lipoproteins (*lipo* is a prefix meaning fat). There are several kinds of lipoproteins that carry cholesterol, but the two most important kinds are low-density lipoproteins (LDL) and high-density lipoproteins (HDL). LDL is the major carrier of cholesterol in your blood. If you have too much LDL cholesterol circulating around your body, some of it gets deposited in the walls of the arteries leading to your heart and brain. Eventually, these fatty deposits build up and cause plaque, a thick, hard deposit that narrows or even blocks the arteries (atherosclerosis), or causes a blot clot to form. The result: angina, heart attack, or stroke. That's why LDL cholesterol is often called "bad" cholesterol.

About one-third to one-quarter of the cholesterol in your blood is carried by high-density lipoproteins. Most of the HDL in your blood is produced by your liver. The HDL actually seems to carry cholesterol away from your arteries and prevents or reduces the formation of plaque. High HDL levels could help protect you against atherosclerosis and heart attack, so HDL is often called "good" cholesterol.

Eating dietary cholesterol raises blood cholesterol levels in many people, increasing their risk of heart disease and stroke. Today, most physicians suggest that cholesterol be limited to no more than 300 milligrams a day. This is not as hard as it sounds. A 3-ounce serving of cooked chicken has about 75 milligrams of cholesterol; an egg yolk has about 210. A cup of whole milk has 33 milligrams of cholesterol, while a cup of skim milk has only 4. You can keep your cholesterol consumption down simply by lowering your overall fat consumption. You don't necessarily have to make major changes in your diet. Just eating a little less meat, fewer eggs, and switching from whole to skim milk would be a good start. If you have high cholesterol, discuss it with your doctor. Diet alone may not be enough to reduce your LDL levels; a combination of diet and medication may be more effective.

A Closer Look at Fiber

In the 1970s, two British doctors, Denis Burkitt and Hugh Trowell, were studying disease in Uganda. They realized that their patients suffered from very few of the ailments closely associated with Western lifestyles. In particular, their African patients only rarely suffered from bowel problems such as constipation, diverticulitis, colon cancer, and hemorrhoids. They had a low incidence of metabolic problems such as diabetes, obesity, and gallstones, and they also had a low incidence of heart disease, stroke, high blood pressure, and varicose veins. The doctors also noted that their patients ate primarily unprocessed foods that were very high in dietary fiber (roughage), causing them to have large and frequent bowel movements. The conclusion they drew was that a high-fiber diet can help prevent certain illnesses.

Few physicians would dispute that fiber is an essential part of the diet and that most Americans get too little. What remains subject to debate is exactly how much fiber is the right amount and exactly what health benefits fiber provides. Many of the health benefits Burkitt and Trowell attributed to high fiber could (and to some extent almost certainly do) have other explanations related to other aspects of diet and lifestyle.

Dietary fiber consists of the indigestible parts of plant foods. These fall into two basic categories: insoluble fiber and soluble fiber.

Insoluble fiber. Made up primarily of cellulose (which forms the walls of plant cells), insoluble fiber has the ability to absorb water in the intestines. This makes the fiber swell up, forming a large, bulky stool that is easily passed from the body. Good sources of insoluble fiber include wheat bran, whole grains, beans and peas, and the skins of fruits and vegetables.

Soluble fiber. Made up primarily of pectin, along with mucilage and hemicellulose, soluble fiber forms a gel as it moves through your intestines. The gel slows the absorption of some nutrients from the intestine into the bloodstream and also adds to the bulk and softness of the stool. Good dietary sources of soluble fiber include oat bran, beans, fruit, and some vegetables.

How fiber helps. By making your stool large, soft, and easy to eliminate, fiber reduces straining during bowel movements. This in turn reduces the likelihood of diverticulosis, diverticulitis, hemorrhoids, and varicose veins. By slowing the absorption of nutrients into your system, fiber can help keep your blood sugar levels steady—a boon to diabetics. Soluble fiber can help lower your blood cholesterol levels by binding bile acids and increasing the elimination of cholesterol in the feces. It's also possible that a diet high in fiber could lower your risk of cancer of the colon, although there is still no definitive evidence for this. People who eat a high-fiber diet generally eat less fat, so it's hard to know exactly which factor is responsible.

How much fiber is enough? The average American adult eats about 10 grams of dietary fiber a day. Most doctors would suggest that 20 to 30 grams a day is a good idea. Add fiber to your diet gradually by slowly increasing the amount of fresh or lightly cooked fruits and vegetables, whole grain foods, and beans you eat. You can easily get 20 grams of fiber a day by eating two to three servings of fruit, three servings of whole grains, and three or four servings of vegetables. If you're not used to eating a lot of fiber, you may become gassy or bloated. Add less fiber or add it more slowly if this happens. Be sure to drink plenty of fluids—six to eight glasses a day—as you add fiber.

Antioxidants and Free Radicals

Of all the terms that get freely (and often inaccurately) used in discussions of nutrition, *antioxidant* is probably the most confusing. Numerous foods and nutrients, including vitamins, are credited with having semimiraculous powers as antioxidants. What exactly are antioxidants, and why are they so important?

As you go about the usual processes of living, your body produces free radicals—highly reactive molecules—as a normal by-product of your metabolism. You are also exposed to free radicals if you smoke cigarettes, breathe polluted air, or come in contact with certain chemicals and pesticides. Free radicals readily combine with fat molecules in the membranes of your cells, causing damage to the delicate cell walls. They are associated with cancer, heart disease, immune diseases, inflammatory diseases, and premature aging.

Fortunately, your body has a built-in defense system against free radicals: antioxidants, substances that bind the reactive molecules and keep them from coming into contact with your cells. (They're called antioxidants because most free radicals are single oxygen molecules.) Your body naturally produces antioxidant enzymes such as glutathione peroxide and superoxide dismutase. You also get antioxidants from the foods you eat.

The most important antioxidants are vitamin C, vitamin E, selenium, carotenoids (including beta carotene and vitamin A), and the many different flavonoids found in the plant pigments that give fruits and vegetables their colors. The carotenoids of various sorts that give color to many fruits and vegetables, particularly those that are orange or red (carrots, for example), may be especially crucial. Although beta carotene and vitamin A are two very important kinds of carotenoids, they are not the only ones. In general, eating a diet high in carotenoids of all sorts means eating a diet high in naturally powerful antioxidant compounds.

Fruits and vegetables are rich in phytochemicals, plant substances that contain, among other things, natural antioxidants. Flavonoids, the substances that give plant foods their color, are one important class of phytochemicals. But flavonoids do more than just add color. They contain numerous complex compounds that act as antioxidants and may also have antiviral, anticancer, and anti-inflammatory qualities. So far, over 4,000 flavonoids have been identified, including the powerful antioxidants quercetin (found in onions) and lycopene (found in tomatoes). Research into flavonoids is still in its early stages. Because we know so little about how flavonoids do their beneficial work, the best advice for now is to eat a variety of flavonoids by eating a variety of foods, with emphasis on whole grains and fresh fruits and vegetables.

Vitamins and Minerals

Vitamins are organic substances needed in very small amounts to sustain life. Most of the vitamins you need come from the food you eat. Minerals, such as calcium and potassium, are essential for such important body functions as building bones and conducting nerve impulses. As with vitamins, you get most of the minerals you need from your diet.

The eleven essential vitamins fall into two categories: fat-soluble and water-soluble. The fat-soluble vitamins are vitamins A, D, E, and K. The water-soluble vitamins are vitamin C and the family of B vitamins, including thiamine, riboflavin, niacin, vitamin B_6, folic acid (folate), and vitamin B_{12}. As their name suggests, fat-soluble vitamins are found in the fat or oil of foods. Fat-soluble vitamins are generally stored by the body in the tissues. Similarly, water-soluble vitamins are found in the watery parts of foods. They are more likely to be destroyed or lost when food is cooked. These vitamins are not stored by the body; if you take in more than your body needs, the excess is excreted.

Vitamins are generally found in two forms: preformed compounds, which contain the vitamin itself, and building block or protovitamin compounds, which are converted into the vitamin by the body. For example, vitamin A is found as the preformed compounds retinal and retinol in animal foods such as eggs. Beta carotene is a protovitamin compound, which is found in dark green leafy vegetables such as kale and in orange colored fruits and vegetables such as sweet potatoes. Beta carotene is converted into vitamin A by the body when it is ingested.

Of the numerous minerals needed by the human body, seven are considered major minerals (that is, a typical human body contains more than 1 teaspoon of it). The rest are considered trace minerals because the typical human body contains less than 1 teaspoon of each. However, trace minerals are just as important for normal body functions as major minerals are.

Recommended Dietary Allowances (RDAs)

Since 1941, Recommended Dietary Allowances (RDAs) of vitamins and minerals have been set by the independent National Research Council. Recommended Dietary Allowances are the levels of intake of essential nutrients that, on the basis of scientific knowledge, are judged to be adequate to meet the known nutrient needs of practically all healthy adults.

RDAs for individuals depend on their age, sex, height, and weight. RDAs for adult women vary if the woman is pregnant or nursing. The RDAs take into account nutrient losses due to food processing and cooking as well as other factors, such as occasional minor illness and occasional poor nutrition. When deciding if you have met your RDA for vitamins and minerals, remember to count both the amounts you ingest through food and the amounts you ingest through supplements. (See the chart on page 17 for the adult RDAs for vitamins and minerals.)

Supplements and nutrition. Most nutrition experts agree that people generally can obtain all the vitamins and minerals they need by eating a well-balanced, normal diet—that is, a diet that contains a variety of foods. If you are in good health and eat a balanced diet on a fairly regular basis, you probably don't need foods fortified with vitamins and minerals or vitamin and mineral supplements. However, not everyone is in good health all the time, and not everyone can eat properly all the time. If you are concerned about meeting your RDAs, you may wish to take supplemental vitamins and minerals. Remember, however, that supplements are not a substitute for a good diet. They provide no calories and no nutrition. If you are pregnant or nursing, or if you have a serious illness, injury, or chronic disease, your doctor will probably recommend supplemental vitamins. Doctors may recommend nonprescription supplemental vitamins for infants and children as well. If you wish to take vitamins on a nonprescription basis, or if you with to give vitamins to infants and children, discuss the subject with your doctor first.

Reading the labels. The federal Food and Drug Administration treats vitamins and minerals as food supplements, not drugs. Manufacturers are not allowed to make health claims for their products. The RDAs set by the National Research Council are the basis for the guidelines used in the nutritional labeling of food, which is required by the Food and Drug Administration. Some confusion may arise because the labeling on food packages and food supplements (including vitamin and mineral supplements) gives the nutrition content in terms of U.S. Recommended Daily

Allowances (USRDAs), which are set by the FDA. However, USRDAs and RDAs are virtually identical.

USRDAs are usually expressed on the label as a percentage of the total. The label on a container of vitamin supplements lists the amount of each ingredient in both units (30 milligrams, for example) and as a percentage of the U.S. Recommended Daily Allowance (100 percent, for example).

The measurement of vitamins and minerals can be a little confusing. Only very small amounts of vitamins and minerals are needed by the body. The units used to express the amounts needed can vary from substance to substance. In general, the amounts of vitamins and minerals are expressed as milligrams (mg), micrograms (mcg), or International Units (IU). A milligram (mg) is a metric weight unit that is 1/1000th of a gram. (A gram is equivalent to 1/28th of an ounce. There are roughly 4 grams in a teaspoon; a dime weighs about 2 grams.) A microgram (mcg or µg) is even smaller; it is equivalent to 1/100th of a milligram or one millionth of gram. An International Unit is an arbitrary unit of measurement used for vitamins A, D, and E. It does not measure the weight of the vitamin; instead, it indicates the potency (biological activity) of the vitamin. Vitamin A is also sometimes measured in Retinol Equivalent (RE) units; one RE is equal to 3.33 IU.

If getting the RDA of vitamins and minerals is good, isn't it better to get more? Advocates of vitamins say that the RDA is only the bare minimum needed for survival, and larger amounts are supposedly needed for optimal health. If you take much more than the RDA of a vitamin, however, you may be wasting your money. Excess water-soluble vitamins, for example, are simply excreted. Also, megadoses of vitamin C (more than 3 grams a day) can cause diarrhea and other problems. In the case of fat-soluble vitamins, some of the excess is excreted and some is stored in the tissues. Too much of some fat-soluble vitamins (vitamin A, for example) can be dangerous and can cause liver damage. Excess minerals are generally excreted. Very large doses of some minerals, however, can disrupt your body chemistry and cause serious health problems.

Some vitamins are advertised as being organic, which is said to mean that the vitamins come from natural sources—vitamin C from rose hips, for example. Organic vitamins tend to be somewhat more expensive than regular vitamins. Vitamins, however, are basically complex chemical molecules; a vitamin C molecule is exactly the same whether it is derived from rose hips or made in a laboratory. In addition, there is little that is natural about the powerful chemical solvents that are used to separate the vitamins from the organic source. Consumers should be very wary of the organic claim.

Some mineral supplements are sold in chelated form. This means that the mineral has been combined with an amino acid to help your body absorb more of it. While it is true that chelation can help your body absorb more calcium, the overall effect is not large. Chelated supplements are more expensive and probably not worth the money. (Chelation therapy with calcium, promoted by some alternative medicine practitioners as a way to widen narrowed coronary arteries, is a fraudulent and potentially dangerous treatment.)

Other Dietary Supplements

An amazingly wide range of food supplements, all said to improve your health, is available. Sadly, a lot of money and hope is wasted on supplements whose claims of effectiveness are based on fractured science or simple faith. As will be discussed throughout this book, supplemental amino acids, enzymes, biologic or granular extracts, and substances such as coenzyme Q_{10} generally have little or no real value.

Eating for Good Health

You don't need strange and expensive food supplements, megadoses of vitamins, or weird diets to help heal common ailments and maintain good health. The ordinary foods found in any supermarket can be very effective for relieving many symptoms and treating minor illnesses. A good, nutritious diet can help you control such chronic conditions as diabetes and can help keep those conditions from getting worse. Eating the right foods can help prevent many of the common problems of aging, such as failing eyesight and osteoporosis. Perhaps the most important reason for eating right—more important than preventing or helping any particular problem—is that a good diet is essential for overall good health.

What Is a Serving?

Breads, Cereals, Rice, and Pasta:
  1 slice bread
  1 ounce ready-to-eat cereal
  1/2 cup cooked cereal, rice, or pasta
Vegetables:
  1 cup raw leafy green vegetables
  1/2 cup raw or cooked other vegetables
  3/4 cup vegetable juice
  1/2 cup cooked dry beans
Fruits:
  1 medium apple, orange, pear, banana, or other whole fruit
  1/2 cup chopped, cooked, or canned fruit
  3/4 cup fruit juice
Milk, Yogurt, and Cheese:
  1 cup milk or plain yogurt
  1 1/2 ounces natural cheese
  2 ounces processed cheese
Meat, Poultry, Fish, Beans, Eggs, and Nuts:
  2 to 3 ounces cooked lean meat, poultry, or fish
  1/2 cup cooked dry beans (equivalent of 1 ounce meat)
  1 egg (equivalent of 1 ounce meat)
  2 tablespoons peanut butter (equivalent of 1 ounce meat)

Recommended Dietary Allowances for Vitamins and Minerals

Vitamins

Fat-Soluble Vitamins
A
Men	1000	RE or 5000 IU
Women	800	RE or 4000 IU
Pregnant/lactating	1300	RE or 6500 IU

D
Men	5	mcg or 200 IU
Women	5	mcg or 200 IU
Pregnant/lactating	10	mcg or 400 IU

E
Men	10	mg or 15 IU
Women	8	mg or 12 IU
Pregnant/lactating	12	mg or 18 IU

K
Men	80	mcg
Women	65	mcg
Pregnant/lactating	65	mcg

Water-Soluble Vitamins
B_1 (Thiamine)
Men	1.5	mg
Women	1.1	mg
Pregnant/lactating	1.6	mg

B_2 (Riboflavin)
Men	1.4	mg
Women	1.3	mg
Pregnant/lactating	1.8	mg

Niacin
Men	19	mg
Women	15	mg
Pregnant/lactating	20	mg

B_6 (Pyridoxine)
Men	2.0	mg
Women	1.6	mg
Pregnant/lactating	2.2	mg

Water-Soluble Vitamins
  B_{12}
    Men   2.0   mcg
    Women   2.0   mcg
    Pregnant/lactating   2.2   mcg
  Folic Acid (Folate)
    Men   200   mcg
    Women   180   mcg
    Pregnant/lactating   400   mcg
  Biotin (Vitamin B_7)
    Men   30–100 mcg
    Women   30–100 mcg
    Pregnant/lactating   30–100 mcg
  Pantothenic Acid
    Men   4–7   mg
    Women   4–7   mg
    Pregnant/lactating   4–7   mg
  C
    Men   60   mg
    Women   60   mg
    Pregnant/lactating   70–90 mg

Minerals
  Calcium
    Men   800   mg
    Women   800   mg
    Pregnant/lactating   1200   mg
    Women over 50   1000+   mg
  Magnesium
    Men   350   mg
    Women   280   mg
    Pregnant/lactating   320   mg
  Phosphorus
    Men   800   mg
    Women   800   mg
    Pregnant/lactating   1200   mg
  Iron
    Men   10   mg

Minerals
    Women   15 mg
    Pregnant/lactating   15–30 mg
Manganese
    Men   2.5–5.0 mg
    Women   2.5–5.0 mg
    Pregnant/lactating   2.5–5.0 mg
Selenium
    Men   70 mcg
    Women   55 mcg
    Pregnant/lactating   75 mcg
Zinc
    Men   15 mg
    Women   12 mg
    Pregnant/lactating   15–19 mg

Ailments
and
Conditions

❖ Acne

It's almost impossible to get through the teenage years without experiencing acne at some point. Only a minority of teens (about 15 percent) manage to avoid getting the dreaded zits. Because acne is so widespread and so distressing to adolescents, it's the subject of a lot of myths and misconceptions, especially regarding food.

Acne is caused when oil ducts in the skin of the face (and sometimes chest and back) get plugged up. The oil (sebum) the duct ordinarily produces then gets trapped and forms a whitehead. The duct then ruptures, resulting in irritation and inflammation—in other words, pimples.

Hormones play a major role in plugged oil ducts. Both boys and girls begin to produce more of a hormone called androgen as they enter puberty. These hormones stimulate the oil ducts, making them grow larger and start producing oil. The process often goes haywire, however, especially if there is a family tendency toward acne, and the ducts get plugged up with excess oil. In times of stress, more hormones are produced, which worsens the acne. Many women are additionally plagued by acne flare-ups that coincide with their menstrual cycles.

Despite much popular myth, there is little clear connection between diet and acne. There is no evidence, for example, that chocolate, soft drinks, greasy foods, or dairy products cause acne.

There is some evidence, however, that foods high in io-dine can cause acne flare-ups. Since almost all the salt consumed in the United States contains added iodine, and since many highly processed foods (including junk food and fast food) contain lots of salt, eating these foods may cause sensitive individuals to break out. Seaweed, includ-ing kelp and nori, is very high in iodine. If you notice a connection between eating seaweed or eating a lot of salty food and having an acne flare-up, you might be sensitive to iodine. Try eliminating seaweed from your diet, reduc-ing your salt intake, and avoiding highly processed foods.

Derivatives of vitamin A, such as Accutane, are used to make some helpful prescription medications for severe acne. Often called a miracle drug by grateful teenagers, Accutane is a powerful medication that should be used cautiously under a doctor's supervision. (It causes birth defects and must never be used by pregnant women.) Some acne sufferers find that eating foods high in beta carotenes, which the body converts to vitamin A, helps re-duce the severity of their acne symptoms. Good choices here are green leafy vegetables, broccoli, sweet potatoes, carrots, and apricots. Megadoses of supplemental vitamin A, however, can be very dangerous and should be avoided.

Another possible culprit in causing acne is zinc defi-ciency. Studies in England and in Sweden suggest that teenagers with acne often have low levels of zinc in their blood. The correlation suggests that zinc supplementation might help reduce acne symptoms. The daily recom-mended intake of zinc for adolescent boys is 15 mil-ligrams; for girls, it is 12 milligrams. Some good sources of dietary zinc are wheat germ, organ meats, turkey (espe-cially dark meat), oysters, beans (especially lima beans), nuts, egg yolks, shrimp, and yogurt. Be careful about tak-ing zinc supplements in capsule form—too much zinc can interfere with your body's absorption of copper and other nutrients.

❖ AIDS

Acquired immunodeficiency syndrome (AIDS) is an incurable illness that weakens the body's ability to fight off infections from bacteria, viruses, and parasites. AIDS is caused by the human immunodeficiency virus (HIV). The virus can only be passed from person to person through body fluids such as blood, semen, and vaginal fluid. Most people infected with HIV in the United States today caught it by having unprotected anal, vaginal, or oral sex with an infected person or by injecting drugs using needles and syringes shared with an infected person. Since 1981, when AIDS was first formally recognized, over 400,000 people have been diagnosed with AIDS; of that total, nearly 250,000 have died. Currently, about 1 million people in the United States are infected with HIV.

Because HIV can't live for very long outside the body, it can't be passed easily from one person to the next. You can't get AIDS from touching or being around an infected person, although precautions must be taken to avoid contact with their blood and body fluids. Since 1985, all donated blood has been carefully screened for HIV infection. Today, you are very unlikely to get AIDS from a blood transfusion or from a blood-based product.

People infected with HIV may remain basically healthy for a long time. Eight to eleven years or even longer may pass before they develop the symptoms of full-blown AIDS. With some rare exceptions, everyone infected with HIV eventually develops AIDS. The early symptoms of the onset of AIDS include recurrent fever, night sweats, constant fatigue, diarrhea, appetite loss, rapid weight loss, and swollen lymph glands. In the later stages of AIDS, patients are susceptible to opportunistic infections that their weakened immune systems can't fight off. Illnesses such as thrush, pneumonia, and a type of skin cancer called Kaposi's sarcoma are common. Treatment with the powerful antiviral drug AZT, along with better treatment for illnesses such as pneumocystis carinii pneumonia, has helped improve the quality of life for most AIDS patients and prolonged their healthy periods.

Sadly, there is no cure for AIDS. There is also no evidence that any food can actually kill HIV or prevent the development of AIDS symptoms. There is also little evidence that megadoses of vitamins and nutrients are effective; in fact, in some cases they may be harmful. Most doctors advise HIV and AIDS patients to eat a low-fat, high-fiber diet that includes at least 100 percent of the recommended daily allowances for all vitamins and minerals. Many doctors also advise supplemental doses of magnesium, selenium, and zinc, since the levels of these minerals are often low in AIDS patients. HIV and AIDS patients should also stop smoking and avoid alcohol. If symptoms include diarrhea or weight loss, special nutritional supplements may be prescribed to be sure the patient is getting enough calories. Because people with AIDS are more vulnerable to infection, they must be careful to avoid foodborne illnesses such as salmonella.

Some researchers feel that an antioxidant substance called glutathione could help reduce the growth of HIV in the blood, although this has not yet been proven. Three fresh foods are particularly high in glutathione: asparagus, avocado, and watermelon. Other good sources of glutathione are fresh oranges, strawberries, broccoli, cauliflower, and peaches.

Recent studies in Japan suggest that an extract made from shiitake mushrooms may have a beneficial effect against HIV. Much more research is needed, however, and there is no evidence that just eating mushrooms will help. An extract from another mushroom, somastatin, may help improve the immune function of AIDS patients, but again, the research is very preliminary.

❖ Alcoholism

If alcohol is causing a problem for you in any part of your life, you are an alcoholic even if you don't think you drink very much. You're very far from alone. There are an estimated ten million alcoholics in the United States. Alcoholics are both physically and psychologically dependent on alcohol. They repeatedly consume alcohol to excess and to the detriment of their physical health and social relationships.

A simple way to tell if you have an alcohol problem is to take the CAGE test. Ask yourself these questions:

- Have you ever felt a need to Cut down on drinking?
- Do you become Annoyed when someone criticizes your drinking?
- Do you feel Guilty about drinking?
- Do you need an Eye-opener in the morning?

If you answered yes to one question, you may be headed toward alcoholism. If you answered yes to two or more questions, you probably are an alcoholic.

Excessive drinking has a damaging effect on many parts of the body. Alcoholism can cause chronic gastritis, pancreatitis, and weaken and damage the muscular tissue of the heart (cardiomyopathy). It can cause impotence in men; women who drink during pregnancy may cause birth defects in the fetus. Virtually all alcoholics eventually suffer cirrhosis of the liver. Alcohol is also a major cause of death and injuries due to accidents. About half of all traffic accidents, for example, involve alcohol.

Because alcoholics often substitute alcohol for food, they consume a lot of calories but get little nutrition. Alcoholics often suffer from overall malnutrition, in part because alcohol depresses the appetite and in part because alcohol interferes with the body's ability to digest and absorb food. Alcoholics often suffer from serious vitamin C and vitamin B (particularly thiamine and B_{12}) deficiencies. Vitamin B_{12}, for example, is found in meat, fish, eggs, and dairy products, but heavy drinkers are unlikely to eat enough of any of these foods.

Alcohol can also cause hypoglycemia, a sudden sharp drop in the level of sugar in the blood. A few hours after a period of heavy drinking, the drinker feels suddenly dizzy, weak, and confused, and very hungry. Eating something sweet such as a jelly doughnut, cookies, or a candy bar can relieve the symptoms. These foods, like alcohol, have a lot of calories but little nutrition.

Alcoholics often have a deficiency of zinc, magnesium, and potassium. Experimental work with laboratory animals suggests that zinc deficiency due to excess alcohol consumption may trigger an increased desire for even more alcohol. When the lab animals were fed a diet high in zinc, their craving for alcohol ceased. So far, however, there is no evidence that a zinc deficiency in humans causes or affects alcoholism.

As long as an alcoholic continues to drink, he or she will continue to have health and nutrition problems. The first step in dealing with the nutritional problems of alcoholism is to stop drinking. Recovering alcoholics who have quit drinking are usually advised to eat a low-fat, high-calorie diet that is also high in vitamins and minerals. Vitamin supplements can be very helpful during the recovery period. The good news is that giving up alcohol will often dramatically improve some health problems. Someone with cirrhosis of the liver, for example, can often recover well if he or she stops drinking and eats a good diet that has the right amount of protein and carbohydrates and is low in fat and salt. Because too much or too little protein in the diet can affect the recovering liver, medical supervision is a good idea.

❖ Allergies

An allergy is an abnormal sensitivity to a substance, such as pollen, that most people ordinarily tolerate. An allergic reaction occurs when the body's natural defense system mistakenly identifies a substance (called an allergen) as harmful. In an attempt to protect the body, the defense system overreacts and produces chemicals in the blood that then produce allergic symptoms such as runny nose, sneezing, itching, hives, or rashes.

Allergic reactions can vary considerably in their causes and effects. Respiratory allergies include hay fever (allergic rhinitis) and asthma. Common skin allergies include eczema (atopic dermatitis), hives (urticaria), and contact dermatitis. Food allergies, particularly to fish, eggs, milk, nuts, and wheat, are fairly common in young children and are often outgrown after age three.

In many cases, changes in diet can have a positive effect on allergic symptoms. Avoiding known food allergens, for instance, is generally the best way to cope with food allergies. Some researchers believe that the symptoms of hay fever can be reduced by eating yogurt; onions are also thought to have a beneficial effect. For more information about how specific foods can help allergies, see the sections on Asthma; Celiac Disease; Eczema; Food Allergies; Hay Fever; Hives.

❖ Alzheimer's Disease

Alzheimer's Disease (AD) is a progressive, degenerative disease that attacks the brain and results in impaired memory, thinking, and behavior. It is the most common cause of dementia in older people. Early symptoms of Alzheimer's include mild forgetfulness and confusion. As the disease progresses, confusion and the inability to carry out everyday tasks develops; later symptoms may include behavioral and personality changes, including aggressive acts and aimless wandering. In the end, the Alzheimer's patient may require total care.

Some four million people in the United States—including former president Ronald Reagan—now suffer from Alzheimer's disease. Because the population is aging, an estimated fourteen million Americans will have AD by the year 2050. A recent study estimated that the overall cost of caring for one person with Alzheimer's disease is $47,000 a year.

Symptoms of AD usually begin to occur after age sixty-five. The risk of Alzheimer's increases steadily with age. As many as 3 percent of all people aged sixty-five to seventy-four have Alzheimer's disease; some researchers feel that as many as half of all people over age eighty-five have the disease. Most people with AD live for eight to twenty years after diagnosis.

Alzheimer's disease is named after Dr. Alois Alzheimer, the German psychiatrist who first described the condition in 1906. Dr. Alzheimer examined the brain tissue of a woman who had died of an unusual mental illness. He found abnormal deposits (plaques) and tangled bundles of nerve fibers. Plaques and tangles are now recognized as the characteristic abnormalities of Alzheimer's disease. In addition, victims of Alzheimer's disease have reduced amounts of the neurotransmitter chemicals vital for relaying complex messages among the nerve cells of the brain. Alzheimer's disease can be difficult to diagnose because other, treatable conditions such as a brain tumor can cause similar symptoms. Unfortunately, there is as yet no single diagnostic test for Alzheimer's disease.

Could aluminum cause Alzheimer's disease? Because concentrations of aluminum have been found in the brain plaques of some deceased AD patients, some researchers in the 1980s warned against the use of aluminum cookware. Later research, however, has shown no evidence that aluminum—the third most common element on earth—causes Alzheimer's disease. Likewise, avoiding aluminum will not protect you from getting Alzheimer's disease.

People with AD have low levels of a neurotransmitter called acetylcholine, which contains a substance related to vitamin B called choline. Since lecithin is a dietary source of choline, supplementing the diet of Alzheimer's patients with lecithin may be helpful in the early stages of the disease. So far, however, firm evidence is lacking.

Good nutrition is a problem for AD patients. As the disease progresses, patients often can't sense that they are hungry or full; they may forget that they have just eaten; and they may have difficulty feeding themselves because they can't remember how, are confused or agitated, or have trouble chewing and swallowing. Poor nutrition can lead to weight loss or weight gain, anemia, and to bowel and bladder problems.

Caregivers can take some positive steps to help the AD patient eat well. Steps that are often recommended include:

- Be patient and consistent.
- Prepare food for easier eating. Cut food into bite-sized or finger-food pieces. Offer several smaller meals a day instead of three main meals.
- Use soft foods if the patient has trouble chewing or swallowing. Serve thick liquids such as milkshakes and fruit nectars.
- Try to make mealtime calm and comfortable; try to reduce mealtime confusion.
- Learn the Heimlich maneuver in case the patient chokes.

Many advanced Alzheimer's patients are deficient in vitamin B_{12} and other nutrients, but whether this is cause or effect remains unknown. The fact is that there is little evidence to link Alzheimer's disease with dietary factors.

Coping with a loved one who suffers from Alzheimer's disease is an exhausting, emotionally draining task that can impose severe physical and financial burdens on you. You are not alone—help of many kinds is available from:

Alzheimer's Association
919 North Michigan Avenue
Chicago, IL 60611-1676
800/272-3900

❖ Anemia

Anemia occurs when your red blood cells don't have enough hemoglobin, a protein that carries oxygen to your body. Your body is then starved of oxygen, and you feel tired, are short of breath, and may have a fast heartbeat.

Anemia can be caused by a deficiency of vitamin B_{12} or folic acid; deficiencies of vitamin C, vitamin B_6, and copper can also contribute to anemia. The most common cause, however, is a shortage of iron in your blood. You need iron to make hemoglobin. Iron-deficiency anemia can be caused by a lack of iron in the diet (especially if you diet a lot), by pregnancy, or by blood loss. Women lose blood every month during menstruation; women who have very heavy periods can become anemic. Another common cause of blood loss is internal bleeding from an ulcer, ulcerative colitis, or cancer. If blood loss is the cause of your anemia, it is extremely important for your doctor to find out why and treat the underlying problem.

Iron-deficiency anemia can be prevented and treated with a diet that is rich in iron and other nutrients. However, only about 10 percent of the iron in foods is actually absorbed by the body, so serious cases of iron-deficiency anemia may need treatment with supplemental iron pills. The recommended daily allowance of iron for an adult woman age eleven to fifty is 15 milligrams; for women over age fifty it is 10 milligrams. Pregnant and nursing women need 30 milligrams of iron a day.

Foods high in iron include liver and other meats, seafood, dried fruits, nuts, beans (especially lima beans), green leafy vegetables such as broccoli and kale, blackstrap molasses, and whole grains. Adding vitamin C from fresh fruits and vegetables to your diet will help your body absorb iron better from food. Some foods can block the absorption of iron by the body. Try to avoid coffee, tea, egg yolks, milk, and soy protein.

A diet with inadequate vitamin B_{12} or folic acid causes megaloblastic anemia. In this form of anemia, the red blood cells are large, fragile, and low in number. The effect is the same: your body is starved of oxygen. It's easy to get enough vitamin B_{12} in the diet. It's found in animal foods such as lean meats, poultry, fish, milk, cheese, and eggs. (Strict vegetarians who eat no dairy products or eggs can get their vitamin B_{12} from fermented soybean foods such as miso.) The recommended daily allowance of vitamin B_{12} for an adult is 2 micrograms. One egg contains about 0.75 micrograms of vitamin B_{12}, while a cup of nonfat milk has 0.95 micrograms.

Folic acid (folete), which works in concert with vitamin B_{12} in the body, is found in many dietary sources, including leafy dark green vegetables (kale, spinach, romaine lettuce, and the like), liver, orange juice, avocados, beets, and broccoli. Brewer's yeast is another good source. The recommended daily allowance of folic acid for an adult is 400 micrograms, but it is twice as much for women who are planning pregnancy, are pregnant, or are nursing. (See the section on Pregnancy for more information about folic acid.)

❖ Angina

Angina pectoris is a dull, constricting pain in the center of the chest that occurs when the heart is temporarily starved of oxygen. Angina is a symptom of an underlying disease that reduces the supply of oxygen to your heart. Most commonly, it is caused by coronary artery disease (see the section on Atherosclerosis), although high blood pressure, anemia, hyperthyroidism, and some other conditions can also cause angina.

Ordinarily, the arteries that supply oxygen-rich blood to your heart can easily handle any increased demand due to exercise, cold temperature, emotions, and so on. If the arteries are constricted or partially blocked, however, the heart muscle doesn't get the oxygen it needs. The result is angina. The pain usually goes away as the demand for oxygen lessens. Angina caused by exercise, for example, will almost always quickly go away when you stop.

Angina is quite common, especially in men over the age of thirty. Because it is usually a sign of heart disease, it should be taken seriously. See your doctor as soon as possible if you experience anginalike symptoms, even if they last for only a few minutes. If you have angina and the symptoms are getting worse, see your doctor at once—you could be at serious risk of a heart attack.

Diet and lifestyle changes can have a beneficial effect on angina. If you smoke, stop. Cut back on alcohol or eliminate it altogether. If you are overweight, discuss a weight-loss plan with your doctor, In general, most physicians recommend a low-salt, low-fat, high-fiber diet and moderate exercise for angina patients, along with appropriate medication.

Some researchers believe that angina may be linked to low levels of the antioxidants vitamin C, vitamin E, and beta carotene (the precursor to vitamin A), and to low levels of the fatty acid omega-3. Eating foods that are high in these nutrients, therefore, could help reduce angina symptoms. Vitamin C is found abundantly in fresh fruits and vegetables, while beta carotene is found in orange, dark yellow, and leafy dark green fruits and vegetables. Good dietary sources of vitamin E include vegetable oils, seeds, nuts, and wheat germ. Omega-3 is found in fatty fishes such as tuna and mackerel.

❖ Anorexia Nervosa

Anorexia nervosa, a refusal to eat that leads to severe weight loss, usually begins during the teenage years. Anorexia is common in America, especially among girls (only about 6 percent of anorexics are boys). Estimates of its occurrence vary, but approximately one in every one hundred to two hundred girls between the ages of twelve and eighteen will become anorexic.

Anorexics have a distorted view of the world and of themselves. They feel that their bodies are too fat, even when they have lost more than 25 percent of their body weight. Anorexics become obsessed with losing weight, often starving themselves down to only seventy or eighty pounds. They also often become obsessed about physical fitness and exercise compulsively.

Anorexia can have serious complications. Some 10 to 15 percent of anorexics die from starvation or related complications such as heart or kidney failure. Another 2 to 3 percent commit suicide.

Although the roots of anorexia are almost always psychological, some studies suggest that a severe deficiency of zinc may cause or worsen the problem. The symptoms of zinc deficiency are similar to those of anorexia: weight loss, depression, loss of appetite, failure to menstruate, and changes in the perception of taste and smell.

Since the best dietary sources of zinc are meat, fish, and shellfish, vegetarians and vegans sometimes have zinc deficiencies, and many anorexic girls are vegetarians. Some researchers feel that as these girls eat less and less, their zinc deficiency increases, making their eating disorder even worse.

The recommended daily allowance of zinc is 12 milligrams a day for women. In addition to lean meat, poultry, fish, and shellfish, some other good dietary sources of zinc are oatmeal, whole wheat bread, peas, lima beans, egg yolks, brewer's yeast, wheat germ, milk, and yogurt.

❖ Anxiety

Everyday life is full of stress: major, minor, and in between. Anxiety—a feeling of tenseness or apprehension, often accompanied by racing thoughts, sweaty palms, and elevated heartbeat—is a normal response to major stress. It's your body's way of alerting you to danger. Sometimes, however, anxiety gets out of control. You feel vaguely worried or fearful for no obvious reason; sometimes the anxiety escalates into an overwhelming sense of dread and fear. Real physical symptoms accompany anxiety: tense muscles, shortness of breath, rapid heartbeat, dry mouth, inability to concentrate, and insomnia are the usual signs.

Anxiety often responds well to changes in lifestyle and diet. Relaxation techniques such as yoga, biofeedback, and deep breathing can help you control the symptoms. Regular exercise also helps reduce anxiety by giving you a feeling of well-being. Reduce or eliminate alcohol from your diet, and eliminate any substance abuse. Alcohol and drugs may be temporarily relaxing, but in the long run they make you even more anxious and depressed.

Eliminating caffeine from your diet is probably the easiest and most important step you can take to help reduce anxiety. Caffeine is a powerful stimulant that is found in coffee, tea, many soft drinks (even the ones that aren't cola flavored), and chocolate. It is also an ingredient in many over-the-counter medications such as diet pills and cold and cough medicines.

Another good way to help reduce anxiety is to eat something high in carbohydrates or sugar. These foods have a sedative effect that can help you calm down. For mild anxiety, try eating complex carbohydrates such as potatoes, pasta, bread, rice, or beans. You'll probably start to feel better within an hour. Eating something sweetened with sugar or honey can help calm you even faster.

❖ Arthritis

The word *arthritis* literally means joint inflammation. In general, it refers to a family of more than a hundred rheumatic diseases that affect not only the joints but also other connective tissues of the body. The two most common forms of arthritis are osteoarthritis and rheumatoid arthritis. Other forms include gout, lupus, and juvenile arthritis. All together, the various forms of arthritis affect 37 million Americans (1 out of 7), including some 200,000 children.

Osteoarthritis

Osteoarthritis, also sometimes called degenerative arthritis, is the most common form of arthritis—nearly sixteen million Americans suffer from it. Osteoarthritis occurs when the smooth layers of cartilage that act as a pad between the bones in a joint become thin, frayed, worn, or pitted. This abnormal degeneration of the cartilage causes pain, swelling, stiffness, and limited movement in the affected joints. Why this happens is still unknown. For some people, the risk of osteoarthritis is hereditary. In most people, it is related to age. Years of wear and tear on the joints, especially weight-bearing joints such as the hips and knees, lead to osteoarthritis. Not all older people develop osteoarthritis, however, and many younger people and athletes do. Osteoarthritis can be episodic. Periods of discomfort are often followed by relatively symptomless stretches of time.

Osteoarthritis tends to get worse over the long term. There is no cure, but the disease can be controlled by lifestyle and diet changes along with medication where appropriate. The first line of defense against arthritis is the nonsteroidal anti-inflammatory drugs (NSAIDs). These drugs, which include aspirin and ibuprofen, block the release of prostaglandins by the body. Since prostaglandins trigger inflammation, these drugs help reduce pain, swelling, and stiffness.

Physicians agree that it is important for people with osteoarthritis to stay as active as possible, If your joints hurt, your natural tendency is to stay off them. This can lead to weakened and stiff muscles, however, and your range of motion can be even further restricted. This in turn makes it even harder to get around, causes more pain in the joints, and deepens the discomfort cycle. Small amounts of exercise throughout the day, with rest periods in between, can help lessen symptoms. Exercises that don't strain the joints are best. One of the best forms is movement in a swimming pool, because much of your body's weight is supported by the water. Water exercise (aquacise) programs designed for arthritic people are often offered at community centers with swimming pools (such as your local YMCA or high school).

One good way to reduce osteoarthritis symptoms is to lose weight if you are too heavy. If you are overweight, your joints have to carry the extra pounds, adding to the strain on them. This can make your arthritis worsen faster.

Perhaps because osteoarthritis is so common and so painful, an unusually large number of bogus treatments and "miracle cures" have been marketed to desperate sufferers. Many people who try the treatments claim they get relief, but it must be remembered that the symptoms of osteoarthritis getter better and worse by themselves. Someone who drinks a cup of cider vinegar mixed with honey four times a day (a popular folklore treatment) might experience a temporary remission of symptoms, but it has nothing to do with the treatment—it is coincidence or the result of simultaneous medical treatment with NSAIDs or other drugs. (See page 40 for tips on how to spot quack remedies.) There is, however, some very preliminary evidence that taking capsules containing omega-3 fatty acids (fish oil) can help relieve the symptoms of osteoarthritis. It is possible that the omega-3 fatty acids, like NSAIDs, block the body's production of prostaglandins. Discuss the use of omega-3 with your doctor before trying it. It can be harmful in large doses and should not be used by diabetics.

Aside from the possible benefits of omega-3, so far, despite many clinical trials, *no* dietary regimen or nutritional supplement has been shown to relieve or prevent the symptoms of osteoarthritis.

Rheumatoid Arthritis

Rheumatoid arthritis is a chronic inflammatory disease that causes pain, stiffness, swelling, deformity, and permanent loss of function in the joints. In addition, sufferers may have general symptoms such as fatigue, weakness, and loss of appetite. Rheumatoid arthritis is one of the most severe forms of arthritis, affecting over two million Americans, two-thirds of them women.

As discussed above, a few preliminary studies suggest that omega-3 fatty acids (found in fish oil) may relieve some rheumatoid arthritis symptoms. Other small, preliminary studies suggest that gamma linolenic acid (GLA), a component of unsaturated fats found in plants such as black currant, borage, and evening primrose, could reduce joint inflammation. However, the amounts needed are very high, far more than could be obtained even by taking supplements. There is also some evidence, although it is largely anecdotal, that eating fresh ginger can relieve rheumatoid arthritis symptoms. If you are being treated for rheumatoid arthritis, discuss taking supplements or eating ginger with your doctor before trying it.

Some victims of rheumatoid arthritis claim that specific foods such as milk and dairy products cause or worsen their symptoms. Others claim that foods from the nightshade family, including tomatoes, potatoes, eggplant, and bell peppers, make their arthritis worse. Still others believe that meat, especially cured meats such as bacon, bring on flareups of symptoms. Carefully controlled studies have shown, however, that a definite cause and effect between eating a specific food and having symptoms is actually quite rare. There is very little evidence that eliminating certain foods, going on a vegetarian diet, or avoiding milk products or meat will have any effect on rheumatoid arthritis.

Arthritis Quackery

The Arthritis Foundation suggests these tips to help you spot questionable arthritis remedies. A remedy is bogus if it:

• Cures all kinds of arthritis
• Uses case histories and testimonials
• Cites only one study
• Cites a study that has no control group
• Comes without directions for use
• Doesn't list contents on the label
• Has no warning about side effects
• Is described as "harmless" or "natural"
• Is based on a secret formula
• Claims it cures arthritis
• Is available only from one source
• Is promoted only in the media, in books, or by mail
• Is sold only by mail order

❖ Asthma

A chronic inflammatory condition of the lungs, asthma causes periodic attacks of wheezing and difficulty in breathing. The airways in the lungs of people with asthma are unusually sensitive to allergens (including some foods) and irritants (such as smoke, air pollution, or chalk dust) in the air. Asthma symptoms begin when these triggers cause the linings of the airways to swell up; this narrows the airways and makes it hard for the person to breathe. The muscles that surround the airways can then go into spasms, which makes breathing even harder. The inflamed linings of the airways produce mucus, which clogs up the airways and makes breathing difficult. In addition to having difficulty breathing, asthma sufferers feel a painless tightening in the chest and wheeze, sometimes very noticeably, when they breathe.

Asthma can also be caused or worsened by viral infections, sinusitis, exercise, cold air, sensitivity to medications, or emotional stress. The symptoms vary greatly from one person to another. Symptoms can range from mild to moderate to severe and can be life-threatening. Asthma is quite common. Nearly ten million Americans suffer from it, including three million children.

About 5 percent of asthmatics are sensitive to the salicylates found in certain medications, such as aspirin and other nonsteroidal anti-inflammatory drugs, and to sulfites, which are widely used as preservatives in foods and beverages. A number of foods naturally contain salicylates and should be avoided by sensitive individuals. These foods include tea, root beer, corned beef, avocados, cucumbers, green peppers, olives, potatoes, tomatoes, and some fruits, particularly apples, berries, cherries, grapes, melons, peaches, and plums. Sulfites are commonly used in restaurants and convenience foods to help preserve the freshness of shrimp, potatoes, dehydrated soups, and other foods. They are also found naturally in beer, wine, and dried fruits (especially apricots). Monosodium glutamate (MSG), another widely used food preservative, can also trigger asthma attacks in sensitive individuals. Asthmatics who are sensitive to sulfites or MSG should be very careful to avoid these ingredients.

Some asthmatics have attacks because the allergen trigger is a food. The most common culprits are milk, eggs, seafood, chocolate, and nuts. If you know that your asthma is triggered by these foods, avoid them.

Given all the above, it's not surprising that some asthmatics report great improvement by going on a strict vegetarian or vegan (no eggs or dairy products) diet.

Although most asthmatics require drug treatment under medical supervision to control their attacks, some simple dietary steps can help reduce the number and severity of asthma attacks.

Because the underlying cause of asthma attacks is inflammation of the airways, eating onions, which contain natural anti-inflammatory ingredients, may be of help. It's possible that quercetin and thiosulfinate, two compounds found in onions, are responsible. Eating a lot of hot, spicy foods such as chili peppers and strong mustard may also help asthma because these foods can help thin the mucus that clogs airways.

The caffeine in coffee can also help asthmatics avoid attacks and relieve the symptoms. In general, people who regularly drink three cups of coffee a day are markedly less likely to have asthma. If you're having an attack, two cups of strong coffee can help relieve your symptoms. This is probably because the caffeine in the coffee contains a substance called theophylline, which helps relax muscle spasms around the airways. In fact, theophylline by itself is a commonly prescribed asthma drug. Don't substitute coffee for your regular asthma medication, however.

Some studies suggest that increasing your intake of vitamin B_6, vitamin C, and selenium could help reduce the symptoms of asthma, but talk to your doctor first. Making sure you get 50 milligrams of vitamin B_6 and 300 milligrams of vitamin C daily, through diet or supplements, may be helpful. The recommended daily allowance of selenium is about 70 micrograms for adults. Selenium in large amounts can be toxic, but getting twice the RDA is generally safe and could help. Grains such as brown rice, oatmeal, and whole wheat are excellent dietary sources of selenium, as are poultry, organ meats, and fish.

❖ Atherosclerosis

Also known as hardening of the arteries, atherosclerosis occurs when excess cholesterol in your body becomes trapped in the walls of your arteries. The cholesterol buildup narrows the arteries that supply blood to your heart, slowing or even blocking the flow. The heart gets less oxygen than it needs, which can lead to angina (see the section on Angina for more information). If a blood clot forms in a narrowed artery, a heart attack (myocardial infarction) can occur. In fact, atherosclerosis is the cause of 97 percent of all heart attacks in the United States. If the narrowed artery leads to the brain, a blood clot can cause a stroke.

It's important to remember that cholesterol isn't the only cause of atherosclerosis. Doctors agree that reducing your blood cholesterol level, especially the LDL (bad cholesterol) count, is very important, but you must also control or eliminate other risk factors. Here are some other steps to help lessen the risk:

- Stop smoking
- Lose weight
- Control high blood pressure
- Control diabetes
- Exercise
- Reduce stress

Unfortunately, some risk factors for heart disease can't be controlled. If you are a man over age forty-five or a woman over age fifty-five, or if you have a family history of early heart disease, you are at a greater risk. That makes it all the more important for you to eat a healthy diet and have a sensible lifestyle.

Cholesterol buildup happens so slowly that most people aren't even aware of it. In fact, even if one of your coronary arteries is three-quarters clogged, you may not have any symptoms. The good news is, if you change your diet and lifestyle to reduce your high blood cholesterol level, you can stop, slow, or even reverse the buildup, and this could help sharply reduce your risk of illness or death from heart disease.

For detailed information about how to reduce your cholesterol level through diet, see the section on High Cholesterol.

❖ Athlete's Foot

The itching, redness, scaling, burning, blistering, and oozing of athlete's foot (tinea pedis) is caused by a fungal infection that lodges in the warm, moist area between your toes, especially the webbing between the fourth and fifth (little) toes. Athlete's foot is annoying, uncomfortable, and persistent.

Although you are more likely to get athlete's foot if you regularly participate in sports that make your feet sweat inside closed shoes, you may also get it simply because you wear leather shoes, synthetic socks, or nylon panty hose.

Good hygiene and keeping your feet dry are the most important preventive measures for athlete's foot. Wash your feet daily with soap and water. Dry them thoroughly with a clean towel, being sure to dry between the toes. Let your feet air for five to ten minutes before putting on socks, stockings, or shoes. Some people find that a light dusting of talcum powder on the feet helps absorb moisture. If your feet sweat heavily, disposable, absorbent insoles placed in your shoes may help. Materials that do not breathe (nylon and other synthetic materials, for example) trap moisture on the feet, creating a breeding ground for fungus. Whenever possible, wear absorbent socks made of natural fiber and lightweight shoes that freely encourage air circulation. Change shoes frequently so that moisture doesn't build up in them.

Adding a few cloves of garlic to your diet every day may help prevent athlete's foot and other fungal infections from recurring. Eating yogurt that contains live, active acidophilus cultures may also help.

If you have diabetes or circulatory problems, see your doctor if you develop the symptoms of athlete's foot. Also see your doctor if your foot symptoms include white, soggy tissue, oozing, very severe itching, or foot odor.

❖ Bad Breath

Occasional bad breath is no more than a passing social embarrassment for most people. For some, however, bad breath (halitosis) is an annoying problem that just won't go away. In either case, simple remedies will usually help clean up your breath.

Most cases of temporary bad breath are caused by what you eat or drink. Pungent foods such as onions, garlic, salami, canned fish, and strong cheeses leave odorous sulfur-containing compounds behind in your mouth. Coffee and alcoholic beverages, especially wine, beer, and whiskey, also leave a long-lasting residue. Brushing your teeth can help a little, but often there's nothing to do but wait for the compounds to dissipate, which could take a full twenty-four hours if you ate a lot.

If you still have bad breath even after avoiding all the above foods, you may need to improve your oral hygiene. Bacteria in your mouth give off the same sort of sulfurous compounds as garlic. Dentists recommend that you brush your teeth after every meal to remove bacteria that could be causing your bad breath. If you can't brush, try rinsing your mouth with fresh water a few times after meals. Floss your teeth daily to remove food particles stuck between your teeth. Bacteria from the particles may be the culprit. You could also try gently brushing your tongue to remove food particles and bacteria.

Does using a mouthwash help? Most mouthwashes contain alcohol along with eucalyptol, menthol, or thymol as flavoring. Mouthwashes do kill bacteria that can cause mouth odor, but the effect is only temporary, often lasting for less than an hour. Breath mints and chewing gum also freshen your breath, but only while they are in your mouth. A better approach for freshening your breath is to chew on fresh parsley sprigs, fennel seeds, or cloves.

In about a third of all cases, persistent bad breath is caused by periodontal (gum) disease. (See the section on Gum Diseases for more information.) Persistent bad breath can be a symptom of more serious health problems such as diabetes, cirrhosis of the liver, kidney failure, dehydration, chronic sinusitis, or gastrointestinal trouble. Drugs such as penicillin and lithium can cause bad breath, too.

❖ Benign Breast Disease

Many women have breasts that are naturally lumpy and tend to swell and become tender before menstruation. The breasts of older women often become lumpy as a normal part of the aging process. Doctors call the condition benign breast disease, fibrocystic breast disease, or sometimes cystic mastitis. Why are these natural conditions and natural changes characterized as a disease? Press most doctors on the point, and they will somewhat sheepishly admit that there's no good reason at all.

Benign breast disease can be uncomfortable and annoying, but in general it is not dangerous. In almost all cases, the lumps of benign breast disease are not indicators or precursors of breast cancer, and having benign breast disease does not necessarily mean that your risk of breast cancer is increased. The lumps can make breast self-examination for breast cancer lumps more difficult, however. If you have lumpy breasts, be sure to see your doctor regularly and have mammograms as recommended. (See the section on Breast Cancer for more information.)

The discomfort of premenstrual breast swelling and tenderness can be relieved with some simple self-help steps. A good support bra helps quite a bit, as do over-the-counter nonsteroidal anti-inflammatory drugs such as aspirin and ibuprofen. Avoid nonprescription diuretics. They do help reduce breast swelling, but they can throw off your overall fluid balance and cause more trouble than they help. Ice packs also help some women. For more information on dealing with breast tenderness, see also the section on Premenstrual Syndrome (PMS).

Changing your diet can help improve the symptoms of benign breast disease. Reducing your salt intake can help lessen breast swelling and tenderness. Many women say that eliminating caffeine from their diet relieves their symptoms, sometimes dramatically. This has been extensively studied and never proved, but is certainly worth trying. Remember that caffeine is found not only in coffee and tea but also in soft drinks (especially colas), chocolate, and many over-the-counter and prescription medications.

Some studies suggest that increasing your intake of vitamin E may help reduce breast lumpiness. Adding 400 IU of vitamin E supplements to your daily diet may help. High doses of vitamin A may also reduce discomfort from lumps and cysts. However, the doses needed to have any effect are high enough to be toxic. Many women with fibrocystic breast disease have low levels of selenium. Increasing your selenium intake to 100 micrograms daily could help your symptoms. Foods high in selenium include organ meats, seafood, lean meat, poultry, and whole grains such as oatmeal and brown rice. Before adding any of these supplements to your diet, however, discuss the question with your doctor.

❖ Bladder Infections

See Urinary Tract infections.

❖ Blood Clots

When a blood clot (thrombus) forms in an already narrowed artery, it can block the flow of blood through the vessel. If the artery leads to the heart, a heart attack (myocardial infarction) can occur. If the artery leads to the brain, a stroke may be the result.

Clearly, preventing blood clots will prevent many heart attacks and strokes. A number of well-documented studies show that what you eat can have a big effect on how your blood clots.

Your tendency to form blood clots depends on how likely your blood platelets are to clump together, how much blood fibrinogen (a protein your body uses to make clots) you have, and how active your body's natural clot-dissolving system is.

A number of foods can reduce your chances of creating a blood clot by making your platelets less "sticky." This makes your blood less viscous (thinner), changes your fibrinogen levels, and helps you dissolve clots.

Onions and garlic can help block platelet clumping and thin the blood. A substance called quercetin in onions seems to be one of the reasons; in garlic, a compound called ajoene seems to have clot-busting effects. Both onions and garlic also contain adenosine, which has a blood-thinning effect. Many cardiologists now recommend that their patients eat an onion and a few cloves of garlic (raw or cooked) every day.

Onions and garlic help reduce clotting by blocking the body's production of a prostaglandin called thromboxane, which makes your platelets clump together. Some other foods that reduce thromboxane production are ginger, cloves, turmeric, and cumin. A special type of black mushroom found in Chinese cuisine, the tree ear, may also have anticlotting effects. Like onions and garlic, this fungus contains adenosine. Coumarins, blood-thinning substances found naturally in licorice, citrus fruits, and some other foods, may also help protect against blood clots.

The omega-3 fatty acids found in fish have a potent effect on blood clot formation. Omega-3 reduces platelet stickiness, lowers fibrinogen levels, and improves clot dissolving. Good sources of omega-3 fatty acids are fatty ocean fish such as tuna, herring, salmon, mackerel, and sardines. One gram of omega-3 fatty acids daily is enough to reduce the chances of a blood clot by almost half. A daily three- to six-ounce serving of fatty fish will easily supply two or more grams.

Another food that may help protect against blood clots is olive oil. Studies indicate that a daily dose of about two tablespoons of olive oil can help keep the platelets from clumping.

What you drink can also affect how your blood clots. The chemicals found in black and green tea may reduce your platelet stickiness, thin your blood, and improve your clot-dissolving abilities. Exactly why this happens is still under study; many researchers think the tannin in the tea may be the reason.

A glass or two of red wine every day may also reduce your chances of a blood clot. A moderate amount of red wine seems to reduce platelet stickiness while also increasing HDL (good) cholesterol levels in the blood. Scientists think that a compound called resveratrol is responsible. Since resveratrol is found in grape skins, it is found in red wine but not in white wine (the skins are discarded when white wine is made). If you regularly drink alcohol, talk to your doctor about having a daily glass of red wine. If you don't drink or drink only occasionally, the benefits of red wine are probably not sufficient to outweigh the disadvantages of adding alcohol to your diet, especially if you have any other health problems such as diabetes.

If you are already taking blood-thinning medications or have a history of bleeding problems, be sure to consult your physician before adding any clot-busting foods or supplements to your diet.

❖ Boils

A boil is formed when a bacterial infection of a hair follicle causes the follicle to become inflamed, red, and tender. After a few days, the red lump formed by the infection grows larger, fills with white or yellow pus, and becomes even more tender. Within the next few days, the pus usually bursts through the skin, draining the boil. After this, the boil gradually heals and disappears, generally within a week or two.

Since most of the discomfort from a boil occurs before the boil drains, using hot compresses to help bring the boil to a head can help quite a bit. Place a clean washcloth soaked in hot water against the boil for 15 to 20 minutes at a time, several times a day. Continue the treatment for a few days after the boil drains to keep it draining.

Boils are usually caused by infection from a *Staphylococcus* bacteria, so it is important to clean the area around the boil often with soap and water to avoid reinfecting yourself or passing the infection on to others. Wash your hands thoroughly before handling food, for example. Good hygiene in general will help keep boils from happening and from coming back. Recurrent boils can be a symptom of a more serious problem such as diabetes, so see your doctor if you get them often.

❖ Breast Cancer

Breast cancer is the most common type of cancer affecting American women. The statistics are grim: Some 180,000 women every year are diagnosed with the disease; about 45,000 die from breast cancer every year; over her entire lifetime, a woman has about a one in eight chance of getting breast cancer. On the other hand, the death rate from breast cancer has dropped perceptibly over the past several years (by almost 5 percent from 1989 to 1992) and is likely to keep dropping. There are several reasons for the improvement: earlier detection through awareness programs, breast self-examination, and mammography; reduction in risk factors; improved anticancer drugs; and improved surgical treatment.

Risk Factors for Breast Cancer

There are several well-documented factors that increase your risk of breast cancer:

Age. Breast cancer is uncommon in women under the age of thirty-five. The risk increases as a woman grows older. Most breast cancers occur in women over the age of fifty; the risk is especially high for women over age sixty.

Family history. The risk of getting breast cancer increases for a woman whose mother, sister, or daughter has breast cancer.

Personal history. About 15 percent of women treated for breast cancer get a second breast cancer later on.

Hormonal history. Factors related to your body's normal production of hormones can increase your breast cancer risk. These include early menstruation (before age twelve); late menopause (after age fifty-five); late first child (after age thirty); childlessness.

Diet. Breast cancer may be more likely among women who eat a high-fat diet or who are overweight.

The above high-risk factors are found in only about 25 percent of the women who develop breast cancer. In most

breast cancer cases, however, no particular risk factors—
aside from being a woman and growing older—can be identified. Breast self-examination, regular checkups, and
mammography remain the most reliable ways to find breast
cancer at its beginning stages, when treatment is most likely
to be effective.

Foods to Fight Breast Cancer

Of all the risk factors for breast cancer, the one you can
actually exert some control over is diet. The merits of a low-
fat diet for helping to prevent breast cancer have been extensively studied. Some convincing studies have shown that
there is a high association between dietary fat and breast
cancer. Japanese women, for example, eat far less fat than
American women and have a far lower breast cancer rate.
American women of Japanese descent, however, have
higher rates of breast cancer, presumably because they eat
an Americanized diet that has more fat. Other studies suggest that a higher overall caloric intake, whether or not the
diet is also high in fat, is a risk factor for breast cancer. On
the other hand, no direct link between dietary fat and breast
cancer has yet been shown. In 1992, the results of a major
study of 90,000 women conducted by the Harvard Medical
School were released. The breast cancer rate was no lower
for women who ate a low-fat, high-fiber diet. In fact, diet
seemed to have no effect at all. Another recent study of
Greek women, however, suggests that a diet high in fresh
fruits and vegetables and olive oil has a protective effect
against breast cancer. Paradoxically, the women in the study
had a high intake of total fat (higher than what doctors recommend), but because most of it came from monounsaturated olive oil, the risk of breast cancer was 25 percent lower
among the postmenopausal women.

The Role of Estrogen

Some forms of breast cancer grow faster in the presence
of the female hormones estrogen and progesterone. Many

researchers feel that high levels of these hormones may trigger breast cancer later in life. Obese women are somewhat more likely to get breast cancer, perhaps because being overweight stimulates the production of estrogen. Losing weight, then, is one possible way to decrease your estrogen levels. Another way may to be increase your consumption of cruciferous vegetables such as cabbage and broccoli; indoles (antioxidant compounds) in these foods could help speed up your body's metabolization of estrogen. Other possible dietary sources of estrogen-blocking compounds are wheat bran, beans, and soybean products such as tofu, soy milk, and miso.

Another dietary factor related to breast cancer is alcohol. Women who have more than one drink a day have an increased risk of developing the disease.

Breast cancer is usually treated with a combination of surgery to remove the cancerous areas and chemotherapy or radiation treatments to kill any lingering cancer cells. For more information on how diet can help you cope with treatment for breast cancer, see the sections on Chemotherapy and Radiation Therapy.

See also Benign Breast Disease.

❖ Breast-Feeding

Breast-feeding is a great way to give your baby good, natural nutrition from the very start. But to do that, it's important for you to get good nutrition as well.

As a breast-feeding woman, you need to eat at least 500 more calories a day than usual and to drink lots of fluids. In general, a well-balanced diet that includes lots of fruits and vegetables, whole grain cereals and bread, meat, beans, and milk and other dairy foods such as yogurt and cheese will give you the nutrition you need. Be sure to drink plenty of water or fruit juices. Orange juice, prune juice, and cider are all good choices.

As a nursing mother, you need extra calcium. Five servings of milk or dairy products a day should be enough. Other good dietary sources of calcium are broccoli, kale, and tofu. The RDA of calcium for an adult woman is 800 milligrams; for a lactating woman, it is 1,200 milligrams. If you think you're not getting enough calcium in your diet—and you might not be if you can't digest milk well—talk to your doctor about supplements.

In addition to extra calcium, a nursing mother needs extra vitamins and minerals, especially vitamin C, folic acid, and iron. Your doctor will probably recommend taking a daily multivitamin and an iron supplement while you are nursing.

Nursing women should avoid caffeine, alcohol, amphetamines, barbiturates, and recreational drugs, since these substances can get into your milk and be passed on to your baby. It's also important to avoid most medications, even nonprescription products such as acetaminophen (Tylenol), antihistamines, aspirin, cough syrups, and decongestants, since these, too, can be passed on in your milk. If you use birth control pills, talk to your doctor about switching to a low-dosage pill containing only progestin.

After your baby is born, it's natural to want to diet and lose that extra ten pounds. If you're nursing, however, dieting may not be a good idea. You could harm your health and that of your baby. Lose those extra pounds gradually over the next six months or so instead.

❖ Bronchitis

When the mucus membranes that line the airways (bronchi) leading to your lungs get inflamed, you have bronchitis. Symptoms of bronchitis include a deep cough that brings up yellowish or grayish phlegm from your lungs, wheezing, fever, and breathlessness.

Acute bronchitis is usually the result of a viral respiratory infection such as a bad cold or the flu. In general, you'll feel better within a few days. If your bronchitis symptoms don't clear up within forty-eight hours, however, call your doctor.

Since a productive cough (one that brings up mucus) is the main symptom of bronchitis, anything that thins the mucus and makes it easier to cough up will help. Moist, warm air is effective. Try using a vaporizer or breathing warm steam from a shower or basin of hot water. Be sure to drink lots of fluids. Six glasses a day of plain water, herbal tea, or fruit juice help thin the mucus.

Chronic bronchitis—bronchitis symptoms that persist or get worse—can be a serious medical condition. It usually begins with morning coughing that goes away during the day. If you smoke, you may think of this as just smoker's cough. Over a period of years, chronic bronchitis can get worse. You may get an attack of acute bronchitis every time you have a minor respiratory ailment or when the weather is cold and damp. Eventually, you may have a constant cough and severe wheezing and breathlessness. Chronic bronchitis can lead to emphysema, pneumonia, heart failure, and other life-threatening medical problems.

Although air pollution can be a cause of chronic bronchitis, the chief cause is cigarette smoking. If you smoke, stop.

❖ Bruising

When an internal blood vessel is damaged, blood often seeps into the surrounding tissues, causing a painful bruise. The area may be slightly swollen and tender to the touch, and will turn a dark black or blue color at first. Over a week or ten days, the color will gradually change and lighten as the bruise fades away. Bruises on the shin, scalp, or around the eye, where the bone is very close to the surface, sometimes swell up alarmingly at first. Generally, a cold compress or ice pack applied to the area for ten to fifteen minutes reduces the swelling considerably.

Bruising is a normal response to injury. Bruises that occur for no apparent reason or after a seemingly minor injury can sometimes be an indication of a more serious problem such as a low level of blood platelets, leukemia, hemophilia, or AIDS. If you bruise more easily or frequently than normal, or if your bruises seem to last a long time, however, the problem is far more likely to be medication you are taking or a poor diet.

Both over-the-counter and prescription medications can cause you to bruise easily. Aspirin, blood thinners, asthma medicines, and steroids are some possible culprits. Another possible cause of excess bruising could be a diet too rich in omega-3 fatty acid (fish oil). If you think a medication is causing your bruising, discuss it with your doctor.

The most likely dietary cause of bruising is a lack of vitamin C. Your body needs vitamin C to build strong blood vessels; a shortage can lead to blood vessels that are easily damaged. Many doctors suggest adding 1,000 to 1,500 milligrams of vitamin C to the diet daily to combat bruising.

Other vitamins and minerals vital to strong blood vessels and good healing include vitamin A, all the B vitamins, especially vitamin B_{12}, vitamin E, calcium, and copper. Because alcoholics are often seriously deficient in all these nutrients, they may bruise easily. In general, a well-balanced diet rich in fresh fruits and vegetables will help reduce bruising.

Another possible cause of bruising is a deficiency of vitamin K, which is essential for proper clotting. This sort of deficiency is quite rare, however, and is usually found in people with serious intestinal diseases. Treatment with supplemental vitamin K should be done only under medical supervision.

❖ Burns

Burns are classified by degree of severity. First-degree burns are minor burns affecting just the surface of the skin. These burns are red and painful, but the skin is not blistered (sunburn is a first-degree burn). These burns generally heal in three to four days and leave no scar. Second-degree burns are more serious because they affect the skin surface and the tissue just below it. These burns are characterized by redness, blisters, oozing, and more severe pain. Minor second-degree burns generally heal in about three weeks and leave no scar. Severe second-degree burns can take a month or more to heal and can leave thick scars. Third- and fourth-degree burns are severe burns that affect the tissue layers beneath the skin surface and the tissue beneath that.

Only minor first-degree burns and minor second-degree burns in healthy adults should be self-treated. If a first-degree burn covers an area larger than 1 percent of your body (approximately the size of the back of your hand), get medical attention. If a second-degree burn covers an area larger than 1 percent of the body, or if it is a deep burn, get medical attention. Any burn on the face or genital region, and burns affecting infants, children, the elderly, diabetics, or someone with a chronic illness should be treated by a doctor.

For minor burns, prompt treatment with cold water therapy reduces or even eliminates the pain, redness, and swelling. Immediately run cold (not icy) water over the burned area. Continue until the pain stops—as long as forty-five minutes, if necessary. Don't use an ice pack. Often, cold water therapy is so effective that no other treatment is necessary. If serious burns are involved, begin cold water therapy and call for medical help at once.

Old folk remedies such as putting honey, butter, or bacon grease on a burn are worse than useless. They will keep the heat in and make the burn worse, as well as providing a fertile ground for later infection. If the burn is minor and you treat it promptly with cold water, you don't really have to do anything else except keep the area clean and dry. After a few days, soothe any discomfort with aloe vera gel or vitamin E oil. If blisters develop, cover the area with clean gauze, but don't break the blisters. Do keep an eye on them, however. If pus, oozing, or red streaks develop, you probably have an infection—see a doctor.

❖ Bursitis

Sacs filled with a lubricating fluid are found wherever parts of your body frequently move against each other: in joints such as the shoulder, knee, elbow, and hip, for example. These sacs, called bursas, protect and cushion the area. If the sacs become inflamed and swell up, you get the painful condition known as bursitis.

Bursitis is usually caused by an injury to the joint, often from sports or repetitive motions such as frequently kneeling down and getting up again (housemaid's knee). The best treatment is generally to rest the area and reduce the swelling with a nonsteroidal anti-inflammatory drug such as aspirin or ibuprofen. Some people find that an ice pack on the area helps if it is hot and swollen. When the swelling has gone down, heat from a heating pad sometimes helps. The pain and swelling often clear up by themselves in a week or two. If they don't, or if the pain and swelling are severe, see your doctor.

❖ Cancer

Cancer is a general term for a group of more than a hundred different diseases. In all cases, cancer occurs when cells in your body become abnormal and start to divide and multiply without control or order. As the abnormal cells grow, they destroy healthy body tissue. The number of new cases of cancer in the United States continues to rise every year. In fact, one out of every three Americans will get some form of cancer in their lifetime—and one out of every five will die from it. The most common type of cancer for both men and women is skin cancer. The next most common type among men is prostate cancer; among women, it is breast cancer. Lung cancer, however, is the leading cause of death from cancer for both men and women in the United States. Even though the incidence of cancer is rising, there's plenty of evidence to show that changing your diet and lifestyle now can help reduce your chances of getting cancer later.

In many cases, no one really knows why someone gets a particular type of cancer. In other cases, however, specific risk factors such as age, smoking, obesity, and alcohol consumption increase your chances of getting cancer. For example, 85 percent of all lung cancer patients smoke cigarettes, and smokers are twice as likely to get bladder cancer. Drinking large amounts of alcohol sharply increases the risk of cancer of the mouth, throat, esophagus, and larynx; if you both drink and smoke, you are even more likely to get these cancers. Being seriously overweight appears to be linked to increased rates of cancer of the esophagus, prostate, pancreas, uterus, colon, and ovary; it may also be linked to breast cancer in older women.

The Anticancer Diet

Researchers at the National Cancer Institute estimate that about 35 percent of all cancers are related to diet. Some other researchers place the figure as high as 70 percent. What you eat now could lower your chances of getting cancer, but diet alone cannot entirely eliminate the risks. By the same token, the National Cancer Institute points out that there is no evidence that any kind of diet or food can either cure cancer or stop it from coming back.

But what should you eat? In general, a diet that is low in fat and high in fresh fruits and vegetables. Strong evidence points to links between a high-fat diet and certain cancers, including cancer of the breast, colon, uterus, and prostate. Numerous studies have shown that people who eat lots of fresh fruits and vegetables have lower cancer rates than those who don't. How much is a lot? Possibly no more than two servings a day, although five a day is recommended. The many different antioxidant compounds found in fruits and vegetables are probably responsible for their anticancer effect. In addition to the important vitamins and minerals in these foods, they contain numerous phytochemicals that are potent cancer fighters. These include lycopene (found in tomatoes and watermelon), quercetin (found in onions), ajoene (found in garlic), coumarins (found in citrus fruits), indoles (found in cruciferous vegetables), and many others.

Increasing the amounts of fruits and vegetables in your diet will automatically increase the amount of fiber in your diet. A high-fiber diet seems to strongly reduce the likelihood of colon cancer, and may also help prevent breast, cervical, and lung cancer. Insoluble fiber, the kind found in whole grains and vegetables, is most effective. (See the section on fiber on page 8 for more information.)

Reducing the fat in your diet can also help reduce your chances of cancer. Today, the average American gets about 40 percent of his or her daily calories from fat. Current guidelines recommend that you get no more than 30 percent of your calories from fat, and many physicians believe that 20 percent should be the maximum.

As you lower the amount of fat in your diet, it is also important to lower the type of fat. Avoid saturated fats, found chiefly in animal foods such as meat and dairy products, and in some plant foods, such as coconut oil. Saturated fats have been shown to promote the growth of some kinds of tumors. Polyunsaturated fats, such as corn and sunflower oil, are generally better for your heart, but they, too, have been associated with some kinds of tumor growth. Best of all are the monounsaturated fats such as olive oil and canola oil. (For more information about the different kinds of dietary fat, see the section on High Cholesterol.)

Eating foods that have been preserved with salt, smoke, or nitrites may promote cancer. In general, smoked meats and fish, pickled fish, salami, and so on should be consumed only in moderation.

Good nutrition is very important for cancer patients undergoing treatment. For more information, see the sections on Chemotherapy and Radiation Therapy.

For more information about diet and specific cancers, see the sections on Breast Cancer, Colon Cancer, and Stomach Cancer.

❖ Canker Sores

See Mouth Sores.

❖ Candidiasis

See Yeast Infections.

❖ Cardiac Arrhythmias

The four chambers of your heart work together to pump blood through your body. Their actions are coordinated by electrical impulses sent from a small bundle of cells found on the right atrium. When the electrical impulses don't get to the right place at the right time, the normal rhythm of your heartbeat is thrown off. Minor cardiac arrhythmias are surprisingly common, and the vast majority of people who have them have only occasional minor symptoms. These have virtually no effect on their overall health. Many people with arrhythmias do not have underlying heart disease, and in most cases, the arrhythmia requires no medical treatment whatsoever.

A common heart arrhythmia is called ectopic heartbeat. Every once in a while, you may feel your heart skip a beat or add an extra beat. This sort of minor irregularity is generally harmless. However, it is often associated with cigarette smoking, drinking alcohol, and consuming caffeine. If you get ectopic heartbeats, stop smoking, cut back on your alcohol consumption, and cut back on coffee and tea. The problem will probably lessen or even disappear.

Paroxysmal tachycardia, better known as palpitations, occurs when your heart suddenly speeds up to 160 or more beats a minute, even when you are not exerting yourself. The attack usually lasts for just a few minutes and stops as suddenly as it begins, although sometimes tachycardia can go on for several hours or even days. Usually, the elevated heartbeat is the only symptom, although you might also feel breathless and have some chest pain. The symptoms are similar to those that occur when you are frightened or very worried, so some people also feel a sense of anxiety.

Paroxysmal tachycardia can be frightening, especially the first time it happens, but occasional attacks are usually not dangerous. The best treatment is to just try to relax. Some people say that deep, slow breathing helps. Cigarettes, alcohol, caffeine, and nontherapeutic (recreational) drugs can all increase the frequency of tachycardia attacks, so cut back or eliminate them from your life.

A shortage of magnesium in the diet is sometimes associated with cardiac arrhythmias. If you get ectopic heartbeats or tachycardia attacks, try adding magnesium-rich foods such as nuts, dark green leafy vegetables, avocados, beans, seafood, wheat germ, and bananas to your diet.

See also Mitral Valve Prolapse.

❖ Carpal Tunnel Syndrome

The bones that form your wrist (the carpals) are held together on the underside by a tough membrane to form a rigid tunnel. Tendons as well as the median nerve pass through this tunnel and into your hand. If the tendons get irritated by a repetitive motion, such as typing, they swell up and press on the nerve. The result is carpal tunnel syndrome: pain, tingling, and numbness in the thumb and forefinger area.

The first step in treating carpal tunnel syndrome is to discover the cause and change it. Since repetitive motions are the usual culprit, try changing the position of your hands (by using a wrist rest when typing, for example) and taking frequent short breaks. Wrist splints from the drugstore may help in severe cases. Nonsteroidal anti-inflammatory drugs such as aspirin and ibuprofen can help relieve the swelling.

Some physicians feel that a deficiency of vitamin B_6 is at the root of carpal tunnel syndrome. Vitamin B_6 is necessary for healthy nerve tissue, so adding it to your diet may help the problem. Too much vitamin B_6 (more than 100 milligrams daily) can be toxic, however, so discuss supplementation with your physician before trying it.

❖ Cataracts

The lens of your eye is normally clear. As you grow older, or if you have diabetes, the lens may develop a cataract, or cloudy area. Your vision deteriorates, often becoming blurred and distorted.

At one time, cataracts were a leading cause of blindness. Today, corrective eyeglasses help the problem in its early stages. Later on, safe, simple, outpatient surgery that substitutes an artificial lens for the clouded natural lens can be performed. This surgery is now the most common eye operation. It is done more than a million times a year in the United States.

People who smoke are twice as likely to get cataracts. If you smoke, here's yet another good reason to stop.

Solid evidence shows that eating a diet high in vitamin A, beta carotene, vitamin C, and vitamin E can help prevent cataracts. These antioxidant nutrients are found in many fresh fruits and vegetables. Orange winter squash, sweet potatoes, and especially spinach are recommended for their anticataract effects. There is no evidence whatsoever that any food or anything else can dissolve cataracts.

❖ Celiac Disease

Also sometimes called celiac sprue or gluten enteropathy, celiac disease is a malabsorption problem in the small intestine. People with celiac disease cannot tolerate gluten in their diets. Since gluten is found in grains such as wheat, barley, rye, and oats, this means they must strictly adhere to a fairly restrictive diet throughout their lives.

Celiac disease is fairly uncommon, affecting no more than six Americans in every ten thousand. The symptoms, including gas, abdominal bloating, and diarrhea, usually begin in infancy or early childhood.

Gluten is found not only in grains but in many processed foods, as well as salad dressings, soups, and ice cream, and in some medications. Celiacs must read food labels very carefully to avoid hidden problem foods.

The diet celiacs must follow can lead to vitamin and mineral deficiencies. It's especially important to get enough of the B vitamins, so supplements may be prescribed. Some vitamin tablets contain gluten, so be sure to read the label carefully and choose a brand that is gluten-free. Dietary fiber can also help the condition, so eat lots of fresh fruits and vegetables, especially beans, nuts, berries, and seeds.

❖ Chemotherapy

The use of drugs to treat cancer is generally known as chemotherapy. Anticancer drugs destroy cancer cells by stopping them from growing or multiplying at one or more stages in their life cycle. Because some drugs work better in combinations than alone, chemotherapy often involves taking more than one drug. This is called combination chemotherapy. Chemotherapy is also sometimes combined with surgery or radiation treatments. Depending on the type of cancer and its stage of development, chemotherapy can be used to cure the cancer, keeping it from spreading, slow its growth, kill cells that have spread (metastasized) to other parts of the body, and to relieve symptoms.

Chemotherapy can be a difficult experience. Generally, the biggest problem is coping with the side effects from the medications. Side effects occur because chemotherapy drugs are designed to kill fast-growing cancer cells. Unfortunately, this means that they also can affect normal cells that grow rapidly, such as those in the digestive system, bone marrow, and hair follicles. The most common side effects of chemotherapy are nausea and vomiting, hair loss, and fatigue. Loss of appetite, diarrhea, constipation, sore mouth or throat, and changes in the taste of food are other possible side effects. Only about a third of cancer patients have side effects, however, and most side effects go away when the treatment ends.

Eating well during chemotherapy will help you cope better with the side effects of the treatment. If nausea and vomiting are a problem, your doctor can prescribe antiemetic drugs that are usually very helpful. You can also help yourself get proper nutrition with these eating tips from the National Cancer Institute:

- Eat small meals spread throughout the day.
- Drink liquids at least an hour before or after meals, instead of with your meals. This keeps you from feeling full too quickly at mealtime.
- Eat and drink slowly.
- Avoid sweet, fried, or fatty foods.
- Chew your food well for easier digestion.
- Drink cool, clear, unsweetened fruit juices.
- Suck on ice cubes made from plain water or frozen fruit juice, or try ice pops made from fruit juice without added sugar.
- If you are nauseous in the morning, eat dry toast, crackers, or dry cereal as soon as you wake up.
- Rest in a chair after eating. Don't lie flat for at least two hours after a meal.

Mouth sores are another side effect that can cause eating problems. Your doctor can prescribe pain-relieving medication to apply directly to the mouth sores. Try to eat foods that are cold or at room temperature. Choose soft, soothing foods such as bananas, mashed potatoes, puddings, scrambled eggs, milk shakes, and gelatin. Avoid acidic foods such as tomatoes and citrus fruit, spicy or salty foods, and rough foods such as raw vegetables and toast.

Diarrhea is a common side effect of chemotherapy. Drink plenty of clear fluids such as water, apple juice, or weak tea, but avoid milk and milk products, coffee, and alcohol. Eat small meals several times a day. Avoid high-fiber foods. Stick to low-fiber foods such as mashed bananas, mashed potatoes, cottage cheese, white rice, noodles, and creamed cereals. If you have diarrhea, it's important to eat foods high in potassium such as bananas, potatoes, oranges, and peach and apricot nectars.

If any of your side effects are very severe or go on for a long time, be sure to call your doctor. You may need additional treatment to relieve the symptoms.

Chemotherapy is often given in on-and-off cycles that include rest periods so that your body has a chance to regain its strength. Take advantage of the rest periods to eat a varied and nutritious diet. It's important to get enough calories and protein to keep your weight up and help your body repair itself.

Some medications, including over-the-counter drugs such as cold pills, can interfere with the beneficial effects of chemotherapy. So can large doses of vitamin and mineral supplements. Be sure to consult your doctor before taking any drugs or supplements.

❖ Chlamydia

The most widespread sexually transmitted disease today is the bacterial infection called chlamydia. By some estimates, chlamydia is ten times more common than gonorrhea. And for some three million Americans (mostly women) every year, chlamydia can lead to serious health consequences.

In men, chlamydia is one of the major causes of nongonococcal urethritis. Symptoms include painful urination and a watery discharge from the penis; however, 10 to 20 percent of all men with chlamydia have no symptoms. In women, symptoms include itching and burning in the genitals, vaginal discharge, dull pelvic pain, and bleeding between menstrual periods. More than half of all women who have chlamydia don't have symptoms. Untreated chlamydia is believed to be a major cause of pelvic inflammatory disease, which can lead to infertility in women. In addition, women who have had chlamydia are at greater risk for developing cervical cancer.

Chlamydia can be easily treated with antibiotics such as tetracycline. Many patients report that eating yogurt with live acidophilus cultures helps them tolerate the antibiotics without upsetting their digestion. Garlic acts as a natural antibiotic and can help clear up the infection.

❖ Chronic Fatigue Syndrome

Chronic fatigue syndrome (CFS) is one of the most controversial illnesses of recent years. Some doctors diagnose it often in their patients, while others dismiss the very idea of CFS, calling it "yuppie flu" and ascribing the symptoms to stress or depression. Because the syndrome is controversial, even how many people suffer from CFS is unknown. Estimates range from 100,000 to over a million current cases.

In general, CFS symptoms include severe fatigue, headaches, muscle and joint pain, tender lymph nodes, low-grade fever, sore throat, unrefreshing sleep, difficulty in concentrating, forgetfulness, and depression. There is no test for CFS, but the presence of severe fatigue along with four or more of the common symptoms is now considered diagnostic.

So far, nobody knows what causes CFS. Researchers are looking into viruses, immune system abnormalities, and hormonal imbalances. As of now, there is no proven treatment or cure for chronic fatigue syndrome. There are, however, some dangerous false cures. These fraudulent treatments include injections with hydrogen peroxide (which can cause blood clots and trigger a stroke), high colonic enemas, bee pollen, and aloe vera juice. The best advice doctors can give is to get plenty of rest and eat a nutritious, varied diet with plenty of fresh fruits and vegetables. Some patients claim that eating yogurt with live acidophilus culture helps them feel better overall; others say that drinking fresh juice made from green leafy vegetables improves their energy levels. In some cases, patients find that eliminating wheat and milk products relieves CFS symptoms.

❖ Colds

The running nose, sneezing, sore throat, coughing, and general misery of a cold affects the average adult American three times a year. Colds are generally caused by one of some two hundred possible viruses. Doctors agree that there's not much they can do for a cold: it will go away in anywhere from three to seven days. In the meantime, you can get relief from some of the symptoms with simple home treatments.

One of the most annoying cold symptoms is a running nose. To compensate for all the mucus your body is discharging, drink plenty of liquids. The liquid also helps keep moist the mucus membranes lining your respiratory tract, making them less hospitable to the cold virus. Most doctors suggest six to eight glasses of liquid a day, preferably warm. Try to avoid sweetened beverages and fruit juices in favor of plain water, weak tea, and herbal teas. Soup is an excellent way to get fluids into your system. In fact, the well-known benefits of chicken soup have been scientifically proven.

Eating lots of garlic and onions may help boost your immune system and fight off the cold virus. Eating hot chili peppers may also help fight the virus, and they will definitely help clear your congested nose and sinuses.

Does vitamin C really prevent or cure colds? This belief is widely accepted, but there's actually little evidence to prove it. Even so, many cold sufferers swear that taking anywhere from 500 to 1,000 milligrams of supplemental vitamin C a day reduces the frequency of their colds, shortens the duration of any colds they do get, and reduces the symptoms. Others claim that taking supplemental zinc (in the form of lozenges available at health food stores) has the same effect. This may work because some viruses, perhaps including the particular virus causing your cold, can't survive in an environment high in zinc. Be careful with zinc supplements, however—too much zinc is dangerous. Take no more than 60 milligrams a day.

Colds almost always go away without any problem. Sometimes, however, a cold can lead to an ear infection, sinusitis, bronchitis, or some other infection. See your doctor if your cold symptoms get markedly worse after a few days, if you're not feeling better after ten days, or if you get an earache, facial pain, high temperature, or a bad cough. Also see your doctor if the symptoms are a sore throat with a high fever, especially in a child. The problem could be strep throat.

❖ Cold Sores

The painful blisters of a cold sore on your lip are caused by the herpes simplex virus, type 1. You were probably infected by this very common virus in childhood. It remains dormant in your body for long periods, then flares up into a cold sore when your immune system is weakened from illness, fever, stress, sunlight, or other causes.

Many physicians feel that cold sores can be prevented by protecting your lips against sun and wind. Frequent applications of a lip balm that also contains a sunscreen will probably reduce the frequency of your cold sores.

There's some evidence that a diet high in the amino acid lysine and low in the amino acid arginine can help prevent cold sores. Lysine-rich foods such as brewer's yeast, milk, meat, and soybeans seem to block reproduction of the herpes virus, while arginine-rich foods such as chocolate, gelatin, and nuts boost reproduction. If you have frequent outbreaks of cold sores, try avoiding arginine foods and adding 2,000 to 3,000 milligrams of supplemental lysine to your diet.

Once the cold sore has arrived, you can try treating the itching, tingling, and pain with plain petroleum jelly. Some studies suggest that applying zinc to the cold sore can help. Ointments containing zinc gluconate are available at health food stores. In severe cases, cold sores can be treated with the antiviral drug acycolvir.

❖ Colic

Excessive crying in babies, also known as colic, can be a very difficult and exhausting problem for both the baby and the parents. Colic usually begins when the baby is only a few weeks old. Fortunately, it almost always ends naturally by the time the baby is six months old. Colic occurs in 15 percent or more of all newborns. It doesn't mean that your baby is unhealthy or sick, and it doesn't occur because of anything you do or don't do.

Colicky babies may seem to be having digestive troubles, because they often eat poorly, pull their legs up as if they have a stomachache, have gas, and seem to be in pain. Nobody really knows what causes colic, although dietary factors may be at work. The gas a colicky baby has is probably from all the air he or she swallows from crying so much. Proper burping after feeding may help relieve some of the gas.

Some pediatricians feel that cow's milk causes colic in many babies. They recommend that breast-feeding mothers avoid milk and other dairy products. If you use a milk-based formula instead of breast-feeding, try switching the baby to a soy formula or one that contains hydrolized protein. Warming the formula to body temperature before feeding may also help. If your baby is a fast sucker who takes less than twenty minutes to complete a bottle feeding, try using a nipple with a smaller hole. You could also try smaller, more frequent feedings.

Motion, especially rocking motion, seems to soothe many colicky babies. Some mothers swear by the washing machine method: put the baby in its baby seat and put the seat on top of a running washer or dryer (don't leave the baby unattended if you do this). The motion and perhaps the noise calm the baby. A ride in the car sometimes has the same effect.

Gentle massage also often helps colicky babies. Try gently rubbing your baby's stomach, or place it facedown across your lap and gently massage its back.

❖ Colitis

See Crohn's Disease; Irritable Bowel Syndrome; Ulcerative Colitis.

❖ Colon Cancer

Colon cancer is one of the three leading causes of cancer deaths in the United States. Some 50,000 people die from it each year. Most people who get colon cancer are over age fifty, have a history of colorectal polyps, and eat a diet high in fat and low in fresh fruits and vegetables. Regular check-ups (especially if you have a close relative who has had colon cancer) will help detect polyps or other problems early. Of all the risk factors that can make you more susceptible to colon cancer, diet is the one thing you can directly control.

Numerous studies have documented that a low-fat, high-fiber diet seems to protect you against colon cancer. Why exactly this is true is still under investigation. Many researchers believe that fats release a carcinogenic substance when they are digested in the intestines. Reducing the amount of fat in your diet reduces the amount of dangerous digestive by-products. Increasing the amount of fiber makes the waste products of digestion move through your intestines more quickly. This in turn shortens the amount of time waste is in contact with the lining of the colon, and reduces the chances of colon cancer.

The fiber found in fresh fruits and vegetables is not the only reason these foods can help shorten your odds of colon cancer. Other substances, such as vitamins and antioxidant compounds, may also provide protection.

Finally, a diet that is low in fat and high in fiber also tends to be one that is relatively low in calories. If you consistently eat such a diet, you are less likely to be obese, and obesity is a risk factor for cancer.

How much fiber is enough? What kind is best? Research suggests that anywhere between 15 and 35 grams of fiber daily will help protect you against colon cancer. (The average American diet contains only between 10 and 20 grams of fiber.) Wheat bran, for reasons that are far from clear, seems to be particularly helpful. One cup of wheat bran breakfast cereal has about 25 grams of fiber. Eat it with low-fat milk. Cruciferous vegetables such as broccoli, cabbage, and cauliflower have a lot of insoluble fiber and also high levels of other phytochemicals such as indoles that may be protective against colon cancer. One cup of steamed broccoli has only 50 calories but contains four grams of fiber. Pectin, a form of soluble fiber found in apples, apricots, bananas, pears, and prunes, may be even more helpful against colon cancer than insoluble fiber. (See the section on fiber on page 8 for more information about the types of fiber and their importance.)

Two other dietary steps could reduce your chances of colon cancer: increase your calcium intake and reduce your alcohol intake. People who consume over 1,000 milligrams of calcium daily tend to have less colon cancer. People who have two or more drinks a day have higher rates of colon cancer. Beer drinkers are most at risk.

❖ Congestive Heart Failure

If your heart is weakened by disease or by a faulty valve, you may suffer from heart failure—the inability of your heart to pump your blood efficiently through your body. If the left side of your heart is affected, it will not pump blood to your lungs well, and you will probably feel breathless. If the right side of your heart is affected, it will not pump blood to the rest of your body very well. You may feel tired, and fluid will probably start to accumulate in the lower part of your body, especially your feet, ankles, and legs (this condition is called edema). If both sides of your heart are affected, you will probably have all the symptoms described above.

Heart failure is a serious problem that can be treated successfully with medications that help your heart beat better and thin your blood to avoid dangerous blood clots. You may also need to take diuretics and sharply reduce your salt intake to prevent you from retaining fluids.

Many processed foods, baked goods, and some over-the-counter medications contain salt or sodium. Monosodium glutamate (MSG), for example, is often added to processed foods; baking soda also contains sodium. Many nonprescription medications for heartburn contain sodium bicarbonate. Read all labels carefully and do everything you can to avoid consuming hidden salt.

If you are taking diuretics, discuss how much liquid you should drink with your doctor. A common side effect of diuretics is potassium loss. Your doctor may prescribe a potassium supplement or suggest that you eat foods high in potassium every day. Good dietary sources of potassium include fresh and dried fruits such as bananas, cantaloupes, apricots, avocados, prunes, kiwifruit, orange juice, grapefruit juice, and potatoes. Potassium is also found in cooked dried beans and peas, in milk, grains, and lean meat.

❖ Constipation

Despite the common belief that a daily bowel movement is essential to good health, the normal frequency of bowel movements varies widely from person to person. Some have several movements a day, while others may defecate as infrequently as three times a week. You are constipated or "irregular" only if you have fewer movements than you normally do, or if your stool is hard, dry, and difficult to pass.

For almost everyone, constipation is a result of a diet that has too little fiber or not enough liquids. Lack of exercise and failure to respond to the urge to defecate can also contribute to constipation. Some prescription and over-the-counter drugs can cause constipation, as can antacids, iron pills, and calcium supplements. If you think a prescription drug is causing your constipation, and increasing the amount of fiber and liquid you consume doesn't help, discuss the problem with your doctor.

Diet is the best treatment for constipation. A fiber-rich diet, combined with plenty of liquids, will relieve constipation and help keep it from coming back. If you are often constipated, try to eat at least 30 grams of fiber every day. You can do this by eating two to four servings of fruit and three to five servings of vegetables every day. Add one or two servings of whole grains such as whole wheat bread, oatmeal, or bran cereal, and you'll be up to 30 grams a day easily. A single serving of oatmeal at breakfast, for example, gives you nearly three grams of fiber, has only about 100 calories, and gets your day off to a good, nutritious start. And a slice of pumpernickel bread has about 4 grams of fiber, while a slice of white bread has less than 1. It's generally best to add fiber gradually to your diet. Suddenly adding a lot can lead to bloating, gassiness, diarrhea, and other problems. (See the section on fiber on page 8 for more information.)

Also be sure to drink lots of liquids. Six to eight glasses of any fluid a day will do a lot to relieve your problems with constipation. Plain water—free, noncaloric, no side effects—is ideal.

Another good remedy for constipation is to get more exercise. Walking just half an hour a day can have a very beneficial effect on constipation.

For quick relief from constipation, try a handful of dried prunes, apricots, or figs, or a large glass of prune juice. These fruits contain isatin, a natural laxative. You should get results within twenty-four hours.

A wide variety of nonprescription laxatives can be found in any drugstore, but doctors generally discourage their use. Laxatives can cause your intestines to become lazy, so that you become dependent on the laxative to move your bowels. Laxatives can also interfere with any medications you may be taking. They can cause foods to move through your intestines too rapidly, so that nutrients can't be absorbed by your body. Laxatives such as castor oil, mineral oil, and milk of magnesia should be taken only if your doctor advises you to.

If you really do need a laxative, physicians generally recommend that you use the bulk-forming kind, because these most naturally resemble the way the body works. Bulk-forming laxatives add bulk and water to your stools so that they can pass through the intestines more easily. These laxatives should be taken with a full glass of water, juice, or other fluid. Results usually occur in twelve to twenty-four hours, but may take longer for some people.

❖ Contact Dermatitis

Contact dermatitis is any swelling, itchiness, blistering, flaking, or redness of the skin due to contact with an irritating substance. Sunburn, poison ivy, and nickel allergy are common forms of contact dermatitis. (See the section on Sunburn for more information.) Cosmetics, soaps, and detergents are other common causes.

Jewelry that contains nickel can cause red, itchy, flaky contact dermatitis where the jewelry touches the skin. If you are sensitive to nickel, wear earrings with posts made of stainless steel or twenty-four karat gold. Avoid gold jewelry that contains less than twenty-four karats, since these pieces usually contain nickel.

If you are very sensitive to nickel on your skin, you might also want to avoid nickel in your food, although it is unclear that this has any effect. Although trace amounts of nickel are necessary for good nutrition, there is no recommended daily allowance. Foods that contain small amounts of nickel include apricots, beer, chocolate, coffee, nuts, whole grain breads and cereals, and tea.

See also Eczema.

❖ Cough
See Bronchitis; Colds.

❖ Crohn's Disease

Crohn's disease (also sometimes called ileitis) is a chronic disorder that causes inflammation or ulceration in the small intestine and sometimes also in the large intestine; all layers of the intestinal wall are affected. Crohn's disease is one of a group of disorders known collectively as inflammatory bowel disease. The symptoms of Crohn's disease can often resemble those of other inflammatory bowel diseases, such as ulcerative colitis or irritable bowel syndrome, so reaching the correct diagnosis can take some time.

The most common symptoms of Crohn's disease are abdominal pain, often in the lower right part of the abdomen, and diarrhea. Some patients also have rectal bleeding, weight loss, and fever. Although most people with Crohn's disease develop it as children or young adults, the cause is unknown. The disease tends to come and go, with flare-ups and symptom-free periods (often for years), but most people who have Crohn's disease have it all their lives.

Getting adequate nutrition is a big problem for people with Crohn's disease. Loss of appetite, diarrhea, and poor absorption of nutrients can lead to dehydration and malnutrition. Some medications are very effective for controlling the diarrhea of Crohn's disease; once that is under control, many patients find that their appetites improve. Unfortunately, no special diet has been proven effective for preventing or treating Crohn's disease. In general, a normal, well-balanced diet is the best approach. Some people do find that particular foods can cause a flare-up of their symptoms. Common troublemakers are dairy products (especially for those who are lactose intolerant), alcohol, spicy foods, and fiber. Others find that wheat, corn, tomatoes, citrus, and eggs can trigger problems. Some studies suggest that yeast can also cause symptoms to recur. During flare-ups, soft, bland foods may cause less discomfort than spicy or high-fiber foods.

It's particularly important for children with Crohn's disease to get adequate nutrition; otherwise, they may have slowed growth. Sometimes doctors recommend special high-calorie nutritional supplements for children. Megadoses of vitamins have not been shown to help Crohn's disease; in fact, they may be harmful.

See also Irritable Bowel Syndrome; Lactose Intolerance; Ulcerative Colitis.

❖ Cystitis
See Urinary Tract Infections.

❖ Depression

Everybody gets the blues sometimes—feeling down every now and then is a normal part of living. Occasionally feeling mildly depressed for a few hours or even several days is very common.

For this sort of mild, temporary depression, doctors suggest a simple remedy: a cup of coffee. Caffeine is a mild mood elevator that can often help you feel more cheerful. Some people find that certain foods help them cheer up. Many women swear by chocolate, especially for depression related to premenstrual stress syndrome. Starchy carbohydrates, such as pasta or bread, or sweet ones, such as cookies or cake, are standbys for many people. These foods may cause your brain to release hormonelike substances that lift your mood.

However, when the blues continue to linger or worsen, it's likely you're depressed. A depressive disorder is not the same as a passing feeling of sadness. It won't go away if it's ignored. Without treatment, depression can last for weeks, months, or years. According to the National Institute for Mental Health, in any six-month period nine million American adults suffer from a depressive illness. Depression can sometimes follow from a distressing emotional event, such as divorce or a death in the family, but often it just happens, like any other illness.

Depression has many symptoms that are often vague or hard for the patient to describe. In general, however, depressed people have one or more of these symptoms:

- A persistently sad, anxious, or "empty" mood
- Feelings of hopelessness
- Feelings of guilt, worthlessness, and helplessness
- Loss of interest in activities that were once enjoyed
- Insomnia, early-morning awakening, or sleeping too much
- Weight loss or gain from appetite changes
- Decreased energy and fatigue
- Thoughts of death or suicide, or attempts at suicide
- Restlessness and irritability
- Difficulty concentrating, remembering, and making decisions
- Persistent physical symptoms that don't respond to treatment, such as headaches and digestive disorders

Patients who have bipolar disorder (formerly called manic-depressive illness) experience cycles of depression and elation. During the depressive period, they will have many of the symptoms described above. During a manic period, they may be inappropriately elated or irritated, suffer severe insomnia, grandiose notions, disconnected or racing thoughts, markedly increased energy, poor judgment, and exhibit inappropriate social behavior.

Drug treatment can help depressed people. Some of these drugs have side effects that are related to diet. For example, people taking monamine oxidase inhibitors (MAOIs) should avoid eating aged, fermented, and pickled foods. Your doctor will explain what foods to avoid. People taking lithium to treat bipolar disorder sometimes experience weight gain and increased thirst; they may also have diarrhea or nausea when they first start taking the medication. If your doctor prescribes lithium for you, he or she will use frequent blood tests to make sure you are getting the right dosage. If you lose or gain a lot of weight, your dosage will need to be adjusted. If you have kidney problems of any sort, your doctor will probably not prescribe lithium for you.

Some recent research suggests that patients taking lithium can benefit from adding folic acid to their diet. The daily recommended allowance for folic acid is about 200 micrograms; some patients have experienced an improvement in their depression by doubling that amount. Good dietary sources of folic acid, a B vitamin, include brewer's yeast, green leafy vegetables such as spinach, liver, orange juice, avocados, and broccoli. Six ounces of orange juice, for example, contain about 100 micrograms of folic acid.

❖ Dermatitis
See Contact Dermatitis; Eczema; Psoriasis.

❖ Diabetes

Diabetes is one of the biggest health problems in America, affecting an estimated thirteen to fourteen million people. Diabetes is the seventh leading cause of death in the

United States and the single leading cause of kidney disease; it's also a leading cause of blindness. More than 250,000 Americans die each year from causes directly related to the illness. Diabetics have double the risk of the general population for heart attack and stroke.

There are two types of diabetes. Insulin-dependent diabetes (Type I) affects only about 5 to 10 percent of people with the disease; it first occurs predominantly in children. Because Type I diabetes is a serious and complex disease that requires careful treatment and individualized dietary management, it won't be discussed here.

The majority of people with diabetes—between 90 to 95 percent—have noninsulin-dependent Type II diabetes (also called adult-onset diabetes). This form of diabetes usually begins in adults over age forty, and is most common after age fifty-five. Nearly half the people who have noninsulin-dependent diabetes don't know it because the symptoms develop gradually and are hard to identify at first. Diabetes does have some clear warning signs, however. See your doctor at once if you have any of these symptoms:

- Frequent urination
- Constant feeling of thirst
- Fatigue
- Slow healing of skin, gum, and urinary tract infections
- Sudden weight loss
- Blurred vision.

If you have Type II diabetes, your pancreas usually produces the normal amount of insulin, a hormone your body needs to metabolize glucose. The problem is that, for unknown reasons, your body's cells have become insensitive to it, a condition called insulin resistance. Some people who are insulin-resistant compensate for it by producing even more insulin in the pancreas. Most people, however, can't produce enough additional insulin to overcome the resistance. In Type I diabetes, the pancreas no longer produces insulin. People with this form of diabetes need to inject artificial insulin into their bodies to compensate.

To understand how diet can help people with diabetes, you need to understand how your body uses food. When you eat a meal, glucose (digested sugar) enters your bloodstream and is carried to the cells of your body. Muscle cells use the glucose as fuel right away, while fat cells store it to use as energy later. As part of the process, your pancreas releases insulin into your blood. If your body can't use the glucose properly, it builds up in your bloodstream. In an attempt to get rid of the accumulated glucose, your body will produce a lot of urine; in turn, you will feel terribly thirsty all the time. Frequent urination and excessive thirst are the most unmistakable warning signs of diabetes.

Obese people are at greatest risk for developing Type II diabetes. Physicians estimate that 60 to 90 percent of the people with this type of diabetes are overweight. There are two other major risk factors: having a parent with Type II diabetes and being a member of certain minority groups. Among African-Americans, Type II diabetes occurs 1.5 times more often than among white Americans; among Hispanics and Orientals, it occurs more than twice as often.

Only about a third of all Type II diabetics need to inject insulin. Most people with noninsulin-dependent diabetes can control their disease by losing weight, eating an appropriate diet, exercising regularly, and taking medication as prescribed by their doctor. If you smoke and have diabetes, stop. Diabetic smokers run a much, much greater risk of heart attack, stroke, and other vascular complications. Diabetics should also avoid alcohol. Your liver and pancreas are already under stress because of the diabetes; drinking alcohol can damage these organs. The empty calories of alcohol can make controlling your blood glucose difficult.

Many diabetics find that their symptoms go away completely if they lose weight, even if they don't reach their ideal body weight. In fact, if you are obese and have diabetes, losing even ten pounds can help reduce your level of insulin resistance. The sooner you lose the weight, the better. Studies show that the longer you have diabetes, the less effect losing weight will have.

Diet and Diabetes

The goal of diabetes treatment is to keep your blood glucose within normal range and to prevent long-term complications such as heart disease, kidney disease, blindness, and blood vessel problems. There's no one diabetic diet. In general, a healthy diet that is high in fiber, low in fat, low in sodium, and includes a variety of foods will help. The American Diabetes Association recommends that 60 to 70 percent of your daily calories come from carbohydrates, 10 to 20 percent come from protein, and no more than 20 percent come from fat, preferably monounsaturated fats such as olive oil. Most doctors recommend a high-fiber diet (30 to 40 grams a day) for their diabetic patients. Foods such as fruits, vegetables, peas, beans, and whole grain breads and cereals help slow down the release of glucose into your blood, which helps keep your blood glucose level from getting too high or too low. Water-soluble fiber, found in oat bran, dried peas and beans, and pectin (from fruit such as pears and apples) can be particularly helpful.

Diabetics need to be very careful about the sugars they eat. All types of sugar (sucrose, fructose, and others) will raise blood glucose levels. Diabetics should eat sugars cautiously and only within their recommended dietary guidelines. There is no real reason for diabetics to avoid table sugar in favor of fructose, honey, molasses, or other natural sweeteners, but they must use any sweetener in very small amounts. Most doctors suggest that diabetics avoid artificial sweeteners. Your body responds to the sweet taste by producing more insulin, which in turn can lower your blood sugar too much and make you feel hungry. Sadly, it's probably best for diabetics to forgo any sort of added sweetener.

Diabetics don't have to avoid fruit because it contains fructose. Within dietary guidelines, fruit is desirable, since it is a satisfying snack that also contains fiber, vitamins, and minerals.

The short-term effects of not following nutrition guidelines for diabetes may not be very noticeable. In the long run, however, high blood sugar levels can damage your eyes, kidneys, and blood vessels. Managing your diabetes through diet is not really difficult once you understand how food affects your illness. The American Diabetes Association publishes exchange lists, groupings of food by type and serving sizes. The lists put foods into six groups: starch/bread; meat; vegetables; fruit; milk; and fats. Within a food group, each serving has about the same amount of carbohydrates, protein, fat, and calories. This means that you can exchange or substitute a food in one group for another food serving in the same group or another group. Many diabetics find exchange lists very helpful for planning their meals. The system takes a little practice to use easily, however. A registered dietitian can help you learn how to use exchange lists properly and teach you how to modify your favorite recipes, read food labels, make good choices when eating out, and much more. Ask your doctor or your local chapter of the American Diabetes Association for a referral.

How you eat is almost as important as what you eat. Space your meals throughout the day. Eating five small meals instead of one or two large meals a day can help keep your blood glucose levels steady. It also helps to eat about the same amount at about the same time every day. If you take oral medication or inject insulin, your doctor will explain the importance of eating soon after taking the medicine. Remember that oral diabetes medicines are not a substitute for diet and exercise.

The Importance of Exercise

Regular exercise is an important part of your diabetes control program. Exercise helps your cells use insulin better. It also helps you lose weight and reduces your risk of heart disease. Discuss your exercise program with your doctor before beginning. It's important to select activities that are appropriate to your health and to start slowly. Many diabetics find that a brisk walk of only twenty minutes just three or four times a week helps them lose weight and feel better.

Foods That Could Help

The mineral chromium is a component of glucose tolerance factor (GFT), a substance your body produces that works with insulin to help your cells use glucose. The recommended daily allowance of chromium is between 50 and 200 micrograms. Some diabetics find that eating foods high in chromium helps them control their blood glucose. Good dietary sources of chromium are brewer's yeast, whole grain breads and cereals (especially buckwheat and barley), molasses, cheese, nuts, orange juice, and broccoli. When eaten as part of a well-balanced diet that follows the guidelines of your exchange lists, these foods could help your diabetes. Some diabetics take supplements containing chromium picolinate instead. Too much chromium, however, can actually inhibit the effectiveness of insulin. If you take diabetes medication, you may need to adjust the dosage if you add chromium to your diet. Discuss increasing your chromium intake with your doctor before you try it.

Recent research suggests that the spices cinnamon, turmeric, bay leaves, and cloves may help your body use insulin more effectively. Cinnamon may be especially helpful. Try sprinkling a little on your food.

Do you need extra vitamins if you have diabetes? If you eat a nutritious, varied diet, probably not. In fact, taking large amounts of extra vitamin C may interfere with how your body uses insulin. On the other hand, additional vitamin E may help control your blood sugar and reduce the chances of heart disease later. Discuss the question with your doctor before you start taking supplements.

If you take charge of your diabetes and work with your doctor to keep it under control, you have a good chance of leading a normal life and avoiding complications. For more information on living well with diabetes, contact:

American Diabetes Association
1660 Duke Street
Alexandria, VA 22314-3447
800/232-3472

❖ Dialysis

Your kidneys remove waste products from your blood and regulate the balance of water and chemicals in your body. When your kidneys no longer function properly—either temporarily or permanently—their work must be done artificially by dialysis. There are two kinds of dialysis: peritoneal dialysis and hemodialysis. In peritoneal dialysis, a special fluid flows through a tube inserted into your abdomen and fills up the peritoneal space. Waste products and excess water from your blood enter the fluid, which then drains out again through another tube. Peritoneal dialysis is a continuous process that can take several hours daily. In hemodialysis, a kidney machine removes wastes and excess water directly from your blood. Blood passes from a tube in an artery of your arm or leg into the machine, and then is sent back through another tube into a vein. The process generally takes several hours, three times a week. Peritoneal dialysis and hemodialysis can often be performed at home without medical assistance, but many people who need hemodialysis go to special centers equipped with kidney machines and medical personnel.

Diet is extremely important for dialysis patients. In general, dialysis patients need to be very careful about the amounts of protein, potassium, sodium, phosphorus, and liquids they consume. At the same time, they need to be sure they are getting enough calories, vitamins, and minerals.

Protein can be a big problem for dialysis patients in two ways. They can build up too much urea, the waste product of protein, in the blood, and the dialysis can remove proteins that would normally be retained by the blood. To avoid protein problems while on dialysis, eat high-quality protein at each meal. High-quality protein comes from animal sources such as eggs, fish, chicken, and meat. Avoid low-quality protein from plant sources such as vegetables and grains.

Maintaining the right level of potassium, a mineral found naturally in many foods, is very important for dialysis patients, because dialysis removes potassium from the body. Both high *and* low levels of potassium are dangerous to your heart, and high levels can even lead to death. Potassium is found in large amounts in dried fruits, dried beans and peas, nuts, meat, milk, fruits, and vegetables. It is also found in large amounts in salt substitutes.

Phosphorus is a mineral found in all foods, but especially in milk, cheese, nuts, and dried beans and peas. Dialysis patients need to avoid phosphorus because a high level of phosphorus in your blood can cause calcium to be pulled from your bones. This can make your bones weak and easily broken. Your doctor will probably prescribe a medicine that binds the phosphorus in your blood so it can be removed from your body. Take the phosphate binder with meals.

Dialysis treatment washes some water-soluble vitamins from your body. In addition, patients on hemodialysis often develop a type of anemia due to a lack of vitamin E. Also, the limited diet you must follow could mean that you don't get enough vitamins and minerals. Discuss supplements with your doctor, however, since too much of certain vitamins may be harmful.

Dialysis patients need to restrict their fluid intakes. The reason is that excess fluid can lead to swelling, weight gain, and elevated blood pressure, all of which make your heart work harder. To keep from getting thirsty, avoid sodium. This mineral is found in table salt and many prepared foods. Overnight weight gain on dialysis is due to probably drinking too many fluids or eating too much sodium.

Patients using peritoneal dialysis tend to gain weight because the dialysis fluid contains sugar. Patients on hemodialysis, on the other hand, tend to lose weight. In either case, you will have to adjust your caloric intake.

Proper diet is an essential component of dialysis therapy. To help you deal with the complexities of dialysis, your doctor will probably refer you to a specially trained renal (kidney) dietitian. By working with the dietitian and paying close attention to your diet, you can help your dialysis go much more smoothly. Be sure to discuss any dietary decisions or changes you want to make with your doctor and dietitian before you try them.

❖ Diarrhea

It happens to almost everybody some time—frequent, sudden trips to the bathroom and the passing of loose, watery stools. Diarrhea is a common but usually minor ailment caused by a virus ("intestinal flu"), bacteria, or something in your diet. Fortunately, in adults the problem usually goes away within a couple of days. Eating the right foods and taking some simple self-help measures can relieve the symptoms and help you feel better. Diarrhea in infants, children, people with chronic illnesses, and the elderly can be very serious—call your doctor.

Diarrhea is your body's way of getting rid of germs or an offending food. Instead of trying to stop the diarrhea with medication, doctors generally suggest that you just try to replace the fluids your body loses. Most doctors recommend drinking lots of clear fluids and diluted fruit juices. Water is always good, as are old standbys such as flat ginger ale, chicken broth, and weak tea. Some people find that sports drinks are helpful.

As soon as you feel like eating again, try having something that is thick, starchy, and not too sweet. Blenderized chicken soup with rice, Cream of Wheat, plain baked potatoes (no butter), bananas, tapioca pudding, and the like are all easily digested and won't irritate your bowel further. For this reason, the BRAT diet—bananas, rice, applesauce, and toast—for diarrhea is often recommended by physicians. It's usually best to eat several small meals spread throughout the day rather than one or two big meals.

While you're suffering from diarrhea, avoid fatty or fried foods, sugary foods, carbonated beverages, gaseous foods such as cabbage and beans, and dairy products such as milk, cottage cheese, and ice cream. All these foods are hard to digest and will only irritate your system further. The exception to the no-dairy rule comes when you are on the mend. At that point, eating some live-culture yogurt or taking acidophilus tablets can help restore the balance of good bacteria in your digestive tract.

Diarrhea is often caused by overeating or eating foods that upset your digestion; it can sometimes be caused by drugs, either prescription or over-the-counter. If you overeat, especially if you eat too many sweets, diarrhea may be the price you pay. Once the offending foods have passed through your system, you should quickly feel better. If you are lactose intolerant, dairy products could be causing your diarrhea, so avoid these foods in the future. (For more information, see the section on Lactose Intolerance). Diarrhea is often the result of a food intolerance or food allergy. To avoid future problems, you need to identify and avoid the food(s). (For more information, see the sections on Celiac Disease and Food Allergies.)

Sometimes diarrhea is caused by the artificial sweeteners sorbitol or mannitol, which are often used in dietetic baked goods, candies, and chewing gum. Sorbitol is also found naturally in apple juice, pear juice, and grape juice. Another cause of diarrhea could be nonprescription liquid antacids containing magnesium hydroxide. High doses of vitamin C can cause diarrhea. If you take supplemental vitamin C, try cutting back. Prescription antibiotics can cause diarrhea because the medication kills bad germs but also kills the useful bacteria in your digestive tract. If you think an antibiotic is causing your diarrhea, try eating some live-culture yogurt or taking acidophilus tablets. If the diarrhea persists, discuss a change of medication with your doctor.

Diarrhea that doesn't go away in a few days or that recurs often can be a sign of a more serious problem. See your doctor promptly.

See also Crohn's Disease; Irritable Bowel Syndrome; Ulcerative Colitis.

❖ Diverticular Disease

Ideally, the walls of your colon are smooth. Often, however, small, saclike swellings or pouches called diverticula can develop in the walls of the lowest part and project out into the abdominal cavity. In many cases, the diverticula cause few or no symptoms, a condition called diverticulosis. Sometimes, however, one or more of the diverticula becomes inflamed, causing severe pain on the left side of the abdomen, fever, alternating diarrhea and constipation, nausea, and other symptoms. The inflammation, called diverticulitis, needs prompt medical treatment with antibiotics and possibly even surgery. Diverticulosis is quite common among older adults. By some estimates, about half of all Americans over age sixty have diverticulosis; only about 10 percent of them, however, will ever develop diverticulitis.

Diverticular disease is common in industrialized nations and almost unheard of in less developed countries. The difference seems to lie in diet. The typical American diet is very low in fiber compared to the typical African or Asian diet. Recognizing this, most doctors recommend a high-fiber (30 to 40 grams daily), low-fat diet as the best approach to preventing and treating diverticular disease. If you have been diagnosed with diverticulosis, adding fiber to your diet can reduce or even eliminate the symptoms. If you have ever had a diverticulitis attack, adding fiber to your diet can prevent another one. Fresh fruits and vegetables, oat bran, and whole grain breads and cereals are all good sources of fiber. Be sure to drink plenty of liquids as well—six to eight glasses a day. (For more information, see the discussion on fiber on page 8.)

If you have diverticular disease, most doctors recommend that you avoid nuts, popcorn, and foods with small seeds (raspberries, for instance). Undigested particles can get caught in the diverticula and cause inflammation. Many people with diverticular disease also have trouble with constipation. Your doctor may also suggest that you use a bulk-forming laxative on a regular basis.

See also Crohn's Disease; Irritable Bowel Syndrome.

❖ Dry Mouth

If your mouth frequently feels dry, especially at mealtime, if you seem to have less saliva than you used to, if you have difficulty swallowing, or if you have trouble eating dry foods such as crackers, you may suffering from dry mouth (xerostomia). Dry mouth is not a disease in itself, but it can be a symptom of some diseases, such as Sjoegren's disease. It is also sometimes a side effect of medications. According to the National Institute of Dental Research, dry mouth can be caused by over 400 commonly prescribed medications, especially antidepressants and drugs used to treat high blood pressure. Another common cause of dry mouth is radiation treatment.

Dry mouth doesn't sound like a serious problem, but it can cause tooth decay and mouth infections. If dry mouth causes difficulty in eating or tasting food, it can lead to nutritional problems. Dry mouth can also cause difficulty in speaking, leading to problems with psychological well-being, especially in older adults.

If you have dry mouth, there are number of steps you can take to protect your teeth and help you feel more comfortable. Brush your teeth twice a day with a fluoridated toothpaste; floss daily. See your dentist three times a year and discuss other possible measures, such as artificial saliva and remineralizing solutions, with him or her.

To relieve dryness, take frequent sips of water or unsweetened drinks. Avoid drinks with caffeine, including coffee, tea, cocoa, and soft drinks. Drink frequently while eating. This will make chewing and swallowing easier and may improve your sense of taste. Chew sugarless gum or suck on sugarless mints or candies. Cinnamon and mint are the most effective. Avoid alcohol and tobacco; also avoid spicy, salty, and highly acidic foods that could irritate the soft tissues of the mouth. Use a humidifier at night.

If your dry mouth is due to cancer treatment, see the section on Radiation Therapy for more information.

❖ Dry Skin

Your skin makes up about 12 percent of your body weight; if you're an average adult, your skin covers about two square yards. The outer layer of your skin (the epidermis) protects your body. The surface of the epidermis is made up of dead skin cells that have been pushed up from the base underneath it. In a single day, millions of your epidermis cells are rubbed off and replaced by new cells. Your skin is one of the first areas of your body to show the effects of a poor diet. Be sure you're eating a well-balanced diet and getting adequate amounts of all the vitamins and minerals you need.

If the air that surrounds you is very dry, it could lead to itchy, dry skin. Dry skin is often a winter problem, since heat from radiators dries the air. Turning down the heat and adding moisture back to the air by using a humidifier can help quite a bit at home, but you can't stay at home all day. Instead, you'll have to add moisture back to the skin. An amazing array of moisturizers is available at any drugstore, ranging from plain, inexpensive petroleum jelly to outrageously priced formulas from cosmetic manufacturers. Most of these products contain petroleum jelly, mineral oil, or glycerin, along with water; almost any of them will be helpful. Select the brand that suits your budget, smells best, and feels best. If you have problems with perfumes and other ingredients, look for unscented or hypoallergenic products.

The itchiness of dry skin can be soothed by an oatmeal bath. You can purchase colloidal oatmeal (Aveeno brand) at the drugstore, or make it yourself by grinding ordinary rolled oats in a food processor until they are a fine powder. Put two cups in a tub of lukewarm water and soak for twenty minutes or so.

❖ Ear Infections

Painful infections of the middle ear (otitis media) are very common among young children. Generally, the infection occurs because the child's short eustachian tubes, which drain fluid from the middle ear, are blocked by swelling from a cold or allergies.

The usual medical treatment for middle ear infections is antibiotics to clear up the infection and acetaminophen (Tylenol) to relieve the pain. The next step is to make some dietary changes to help keep the infection from recurring.

Breast-fed babies usually have fewer ear infections, since they receive antibodies to respiratory infections from their mothers. If you're considering breast-feeding, this is another good reason to do it. If you bottle-feed, always make sure the baby's head is elevated while he drinks; otherwise, fluid can get into his eustachian tubes and cause discomfort and an infection. If the child has an ear infection, elevate the head of the bed at night to help fluid drain from the eustachian tubes.

Because swallowing helps keep the eustachian tubes open, small, frequent sips of liquid can help relieve discomfort. Breathing clean, moist air also helps. Use a humidifier; avoid wood smoke and cigarette smoke.

In many cases, children with recurring ear infections also have food allergies. The most common triggers are eggs, milk and other dairy products, peanuts, and wheat. Ear problems often clear up when one or more of these foods are eliminated from the diet. If you think food allergies could be the cause of your child's frequent ear infections, discuss the problem with your doctor.

❖ Eating Disorders

See Anorexia Nervosa.

❖ Eczema

If you have eczema, you have patches of swollen, red, flaky, itchy, or blistered skin. It's a very common condition. In many cases, eczema is caused by contact with an irritating substance such as a harsh soap or chemical. Once you stop the contact—by wearing rubber gloves to do the dishes, for example—the eczema goes away.

In some cases, especially in children, dermatitis is caused by a food allergy. Sometimes eliminating eggs, milk, or orange juice can help clear up the problem. A more severe form of eczema, dermatitis herpetiformes, is caused by an allergy to gluten. (See the section on Celiac Disease for more information.)

Serious deficiencies of vitamin A, the B vitamins (especially vitamins B_2 and B_6), or vitamin C can cause eczema-like symptoms.

The itchiness of eczema can be soothed by an oatmeal bath. You can purchase colloidal oatmeal (Aveeno brand) at the drugstore, or make it yourself by grinding ordinary rolled oats in a food processor until they are a fine powder. Put two cups in a tub of lukewarm water and soak for twenty minutes or so. Another good way to relieve eczema symptoms is with a milk compress. Soak a gauze square or washcloth in ice-cold milk and hold it against the affected area for a few minutes. Repeat twice more; repeat the treatment several times a day.

❖ Edema

See Congestive Heart Failure.

❖ Epilepsy

Disturbed electrical activity in the brain results in the condition called epilepsy. The human brain contains about twelve billion nerve cells, which communicate with each other and the rest of the body via electrical impulses. When the brain is damaged, the smooth flow may be disrupted. The brain cells can overload and give off too much electricity. The result of the temporary overload is a seizure—a temporary loss of consciousness, often in association with motor activity.

Two million Americans—one in every hundred—has epilepsy. The condition can usually be controlled with medication and the epileptic can generally live a normal life. In fact, nearly 80 percent of people taking anticonvulsant medication have no seizures. Long-term use of anticonvulsant medications can lead to low levels of vitamin D, vitamin B_{12}, and folic acid. On the other hand, taking supplemental B vitamins can interfere with some medications. If you take anticonvulsants, discuss vitamin supplements with your doctor.

The artificial sweetener aspartame (NutraSweet) has sometimes been blamed for an increase in seizures among epileptics. Careful investigation has shown, however, that there is no data to support this claim.

In some rare cases, medication does not help epilepsy. Some of these patients respond well to a very high-fat, low-carbohydrate (ketogenic) diet. Close medical supervision is essential to this treatment.

❖ Fatigue

Being tired all the time is such a common feeling for many people that they accept it as normal. While it is natural to feel tired if you're under a lot of stress or if you haven't been getting enough sleep, it's also possible that poor nutrition is contributing to the problem. If you're constantly rushed for time, you may be falling into some bad nutritional habits: skipping breakfast or other meals, eating too much convenience food, snacking on junk food, or drinking too much coffee and not enough other fluids. And if you also smoke or drink alcohol, you're robbing your body of even more nutrients. When you fuel your body with empty calories, your energy levels are lower than they could be. You also deplete your body's stores of essential vitamins and minerals, which could lead to low-level deficiencies that make you feel tired.

It's not always possible to eat a good, well-balanced diet. With just a little effort, however, you can probably eat better more often, and even a small improvement in your diet can lead to a big improvement in the way you feel. (See the introduction for more information on healthy eating.) You could also try taking a daily multivitamin and mineral supplement. Of course, supplements are no substitute for a good diet, but they can help provide the missing nutrients you need.

Fatigue can be a warning sign that an illness such as a cold or flu is coming; it can also be a symptom of other conditions such as diabetes, anemia, or chronic fatigue syndrome. See your doctor if you are severely fatigued for more than few days for no obvious reason.

❖ Fever

Fever is a symptom of an illness or infection. Fever is usually a normal, even helpful, response to the problem and will go away as you get better. If the fever is making you uncomfortable, most doctors suggest taking acetaminophen (Tylenol) to help bring it down.

If you're running a fever, be sure to drink plenty of liquids. Plain water is fine; so are fruit and vegetable juices, soft drinks, weak tea, herbal teas, ice pops, and crushed ice.

A fever over 102 degrees F. in an adult or over 103 degrees F. in a child that lasts for more than a day or so could indicate a serious illness. Call your doctor.

❖ Fissure

A fissure is a small tear or ulcer in the mucus membrane of the anus. Anal fissures are often just as painful as hemorrhoids, and one important part of their treatment is similar: Eat a high-fiber diet and drink plenty of liquids. The goal is to produce a large, soft stool that is easily passed. Once you're no longer straining to pass hard stools, the fissure has a chance to heal, and you'll be less likely to get another one.

While you're healing, try to avoid anything that will give you diarrhea, since this will irritate the fissure further. You might also want to avoid spicy foods during this time.

See also Hemorrhoids.

❖ Flatulence
See Gas.

❖ Food Allergies

Although many people believe they are allergic to at least one food, genuine food allergies are actually quite rare—only about 1 percent of the adult population and 2 percent of children are affected. Many people do have food intolerances because they lack certain digestive enzymes such as lactase; others have reactions to some food additives such as MSG; and others have reactions to some substances such as sulfites found naturally in food. If you already have asthma or allergies to other things, you are somewhat more likely to have food allergies.

If you are genuinely allergic to a food, eating it will cause you to have an immunological response. Common symptoms of food allergy include itching, hives, rashes, facial swelling (especially the lips), and swelling of the hands and feet. Asthma, abdominal pain, nausea, vomiting, and diarrhea are other common symptoms. Usually, an allergic reaction to a food appears within an hour of eating it. The symptoms can sometimes take a day or two to appear, however, so at first you may not realize that your diarrhea, for example, is an allergic reaction to something you ate earlier. Adults can develop food allergies suddenly at any age, so if you start frequently experiencing any of the symptoms above, it's possible that you have become allergic to one or more foods.

The most common causes of food allergies are milk, nuts and seeds, shellfish, eggs, wheat, corn, berries, and legumes (including peas, beans, and peanuts). If you think you have developed a food allergy, see your doctor. It's important to make sure that some other problem isn't causing your symptoms. If a food allergy is the prime suspect, your doctor will probably recommend eliminating all possible allergens from your diet. You will then add the foods back, one at a time, until the symptoms return. You might want to keep a food diary during this period, to determine what you ate when and how you felt afterward.

Your doctor may also suggest skin tests and blood tests to help determine the allergy-causing food. These methods often give misleading results, however, indicating that you are allergic to a food when you're really not.

Once you've determined what food is causing the allergy, the only treatment is to avoid it. Remember that if you are allergic to one food in a food group, you are probably allergic to all the foods in that group. If, for example, you are allergic to shrimp, you should avoid all shellfish, including clams, crabs, lobsters, and oysters. You will also have to be careful about what you order when you eat out, and you'll have to read food labels carefully to avoid your allergens.

See also Asthma; Celiac Disease; Irritable Bowel Syndrome; Lactose Intolerance.

❖ Gallstones

Although some twenty million Americans—about 10 percent of the population—have gallstones, the vast majority don't know it or have no symptoms. Enough people do have severe symptoms, however, to make gallbladder removal the most common abdominal surgical procedure in the United States: some 500,000 people a year undergo this operation.

Your gallbladder is a small, pear-shaped organ about 3 to 5 inches long. It lies underneath the liver in the upper right side of the abdomen. The gallbladder serves as a reservoir for bile, a fluid made by the liver and used by the body to digest food. Small tubes called bile ducts connect the gallbladder to the liver and to the small intestine. Between meals, bile accumulates in the gallbladder. When you eat, the gallbladder contracts and empties bile into the small intestine.

Excess cholesterol is removed from your blood by the liver and secreted into bile. When the bile contains too much cholesterol, small crystals form in it and the excess cholesterol falls into the bottom of the gallbladder. Eventually, the crystals form into gallstones. In most cases, the gallstones are harmless and symptomless. Sometimes, however, the stones cause irritation or even get lodged in the bile ducts. Gallstone symptoms include severe, intermittent pain in the right upper abdomen (this pain is sometimes mistaken for a heart attack) and chronic indigestion and nausea.

Common risk factors for developing gallstone disease include obesity, getting older, being a woman, pregnancy, hormonal birth control pills, estrogen replacement therapy for menopause, family history of gallstones, being of Native American ancestry, and recently losing a lot of weight.

The biggest risk factor for gallstones is obesity. The risk is three to seven times higher for people who are more than 10 percent over their ideal weight. Crash diets that lead to losing a lot of weight rapidly, or losing weight rapidly and then gaining it back again, can bring on gallstone trouble. If you are obese and want to avoid gallstone disease, it's probably best to lose weight sensibly and try to keep it off.

Since most gallstones are made of cholesterol, eating a low-cholesterol, low-fat diet would seem to make sense. In fact, there's not much evidence to show that diet has anything to do with causing gallstones (except, of course, that eating too much makes you obese) or that changing your diet to avoid fatty foods will stop the problem or keep it from developing. There is some evidence, however, that eating a diet high in fresh vegetables, nuts, and beans and legumes can help reduce your chances of getting gallbladder trouble. In this case, it's probably not just the fiber that helps—researchers think it's possible that something in the vegetable protein can block or even dissolve the gallstones.

Women who skip breakfast or just have coffee on an empty stomach are somewhat more likely to get gallstones. So are people who eat a low-fiber, high-sugar diet. Eating a good, high-fiber breakfast every day—a bowl of oatmeal and two slices of whole wheat toast instead of bacon and eggs, for example—could help prevent or reduce your gallbladder symptoms.

❖ Gas

Intestinal gas (flatulence) may be uncomfortable and embarrassing, but at least you have the consolation of knowing that everyone has gas to a greater or lesser degree. A certain amount of intestinal gas is a normal by-product of digestion. In fact, the average person passes gas about fourteen times a day, for a volume of about a quart.

Some foods do produce more gas when digested than others. Beans, of course, are famous for producing flatulence, as are broccoli, brussels sprouts, cabbage, cauliflower, kale, onions, peas, and turnips. If you are lactose intolerant and have trouble digesting milk and dairy products, one of the main symptoms will be gas. (See the section on Lactose Intolerance for more information.) Some people find that high-pectin fruits such as apples, apple cider, blueberries, pears, and bananas give them gas.

Don't let flatulence problems keep you from eating beans and lentils. They're a healthy and delicious way to add low-calorie, low-fat protein, carbohydrates, and fiber to your diet. Instead, soak dried beans for at least twelve hours in three cups of water for every cup of beans. Drain and rinse well before cooking the beans. If you use canned beans, drain off the liquid and rinse well before eating. Soaking and rinsing removes much of the indigestible sugars in the bean skins, sharply reducing the among of gas they can produce.

Don't add baking soda to the beans. It won't help the gas, and it will make the beans hard. You could add garlic, nut-meg, or ginger to the beans, however. Many people claim these spices reduce the gas problem.

Drinking carbonated beverages or swallowing air when you eat can also cause gas. Try cutting back on soda pop, seltzer, and beer; give up chewing gum and smoking. Also try eating more slowly and chewing carefully with your mouth firmly closed.

❖ Gingivitis

See Gum Diseases.

❖ Glaucoma

If you have the eye disease glaucoma, the normal fluid pressure inside your eyes gradually rises. This causes damage to the retina and optic nerve, which leads to vision loss or even blindness. Glaucoma affects nearly three million people in the United States and is a leading cause of blindness. The people most at risk for glaucoma are African-Americans over age forty (African-Americans between the ages of forty-five and sixty-five are fifteen times more likely to become blind from glaucoma than white Americans); anyone over age sixty; and people with a family history of glaucoma. You're also at risk if you are very nearsighted or have diabetes.

If glaucoma is detected early during a routine eye examination, the prospects for controlling the disease and preventing vision loss are very good. If you fall into one of the high-risk groups, the National Eye Institute recommends that you have your eyes examined through dilated pupils every two years. Glaucoma usually has no obvious symptoms until it has already damaged your eyes.

There is no cure for glaucoma, but most people respond well to medication. In some cases where medication is ineffective, laser surgery or microsurgery may be helpful.

Some dietary steps can also help control glaucoma, although they are not a substitute for taking your medication. A good overall diet and regular exercise are helpful; try to lose weight if you are too heavy. If you smoke, stop. To help keep the pressure in your eyes from rising, cut back on or eliminate caffeine, avoid drinking large amounts of fluids all at once, and cut back on salt.

It's possible that taking supplemental vitamin C (500 milligrams daily) may help reduce eye pressure in people with glaucoma. Some preliminary animal research suggests that fish oil (omega-3 fatty acids) may also reduce eye pressure. If you are at risk for glaucoma, extra vitamin C and fish oil could help keep you from developing the disease. If you have glaucoma, extra vitamin C and fish oil could help, but consult your eye doctor first. These are no substitute for glaucoma medication. Good dietary sources of vitamin C are citrus fruits and juices, brussels sprouts, strawberries, broccoli, and collard greens. Fish oil is found in cod liver oil and fatty deep-sea fish such as mackerel, salmon, tuna, sardines, and herring.

❖ Gout

Gout is actually a form of arthritis that occurs when there is too much uric acid in the blood. Crystals of the acid get deposited in the joints, particularly the big toe, causing the joint to swell up and become extremely painful. Gout is almost exclusively a disease of men: over 90 percent of people with gout are male.

The pain of gout attacks can be relieved with drugs, including nonsteroidal anti-inflammatories such as ibuprofen. Changing your diet can reduce the number and severity of your gout attacks. Eliminate alcohol, because alcohol prevents your body from excreting uric acid. Lose weight—more than half of all people with gout are overweight. Most importantly, avoid eating foods that contain purine, since uric acid is a by-product of digesting these foods. Meats, particularly organ meats, are very high in purine. Avoid completely liver, brains, kidneys, and other organ meats; also avoid meat gravies and processed meats such as sausage and lunch meats, since these products often contain organ meats. Fish, particularly fatty fish, is also high in purine. Avoid shrimp, sardines, anchovies, mackerel, salmon, and other deep-sea fish; freshwater fish are usually acceptable in moderation. Foods that are moderately high in purine include asparagus, beans, bran, celery, lentils, mushrooms, oatmeal, peas, poultry, radishes, seafood, spinach, and wheat germ. These foods should be eaten only in moderation; if gout symptoms occur after eating any of these foods, avoid them.

To help dilute the uric acid in the blood, gout patients should drink a lot of fluids—at least two quarts a day. Some people with gout find that eating cherries, blueberries, or strawberries (or drinking juice made from these fruits) every day helps prevent attacks.

❖ Gum Diseases

There are two common gum (periodontal) diseases: gingivitis and periodontitis (sometimes called pyorrhea). Gingivitis is an infection of the gums. As a result, the gums become red and inflamed and may bleed when you brush your teeth. Gingivitis is caused by the buildup of plaque—a sticky mass of harmful germs—on your teeth. You can usually get rid of gingivitis by improving your dental hygiene. To prevent plaque buildup, brush your teeth twice a day, floss daily, and have your teeth cleaned professionally at least once a year.

Gingivitis is the first sign that something is wrong with your gums. If not treated, gingivitis can progress to a more destructive type of gum disease called periodontitis. This is an infection of the tissues that help anchor your teeth into your jaw. Signs of periodontitis include painful, bleeding gums, abscesses, and bad breath. The infection can lead to loss of the bone that holds the tooth in its socket, which in turn may lead to tooth loss. Since periodontitis affects the roots of your teeth below the gum, better dental hygiene won't reach the problem. You need treatment from a dentist or a periodontist (a dentist who specializes in treating gum diseases). Scaling to remove plaque and planing to smooth the tooth root are effective treatments for periodontitis; your dentist may also recommend a special mouthwash containing chlorhexidine. If you have developed deep pockets of infection around your teeth, gum surgery may be necessary.

Although good dental hygiene is the best way to prevent gum disease, diet can play an important role. Because your body needs calcium to build strong teeth, a diet that contains from 1,000 to 2,000 milligrams of calcium daily may help, especially for older women. Good dietary sources of calcium are yogurt, sardines, milk, cheese, and bean curd (tofu).

A steady diet of soft foods tends to produce more plaque, leading to more periodontal disease. To help keep your gums healthy, eat some crisp, raw vegetables or fresh fruit every day. The fiber in the vegetables cleans and stimulates your gums, so a carrot, apple, or celery stalk a day could help keep you out of the dentist's chair.

❖ Hangover

The inevitable aftereffect of drinking too much alcohol is a hangover: headache, nausea, and fatigue. Generations of drinkers have passed along numerous folk cures, but the sad fact is that there is nothing that will prevent a hangover. The only question is how severe it will be and what you can do to relieve the symptoms.

To reduce the severity of a hangover, simply drink less or drink more slowly. Space your drinks out so that you metabolize the alcohol you have drunk before you drink more. Avoid whisky and other dark liquors and stick to clear alcohol such as vodka. Dark liquors get their color and flavor from substances called congeners; these can add to your hangover misery. The alcohol in carbonated drinks (mixers, beer, sparkling wines) is absorbed into your body faster, so you feel the effects sooner and may drink more. Red wine contains substances that can be migraine triggers for some people.

Because alcohol has a dehydrating effect, try drinking a large glass of water or fruit juice before going to bed. Repeat the treatment in the morning. The liquid replenishes the lost fluids; the fructose in fruit juice may also help you metabolize the alcohol in your system. Some people claim that taking a nonprescription painkiller such as aspirin along with the bedtime liquid markedly reduces their symptoms in the morning. Do not take acetaminophen (Tylenol) or ibuprofen (Advil) if you've been drinking alcohol, because liver damage can result.

The headache of a hangover can be relieved somewhat with aspirin. A cup or two of coffee also often helps. An old Italian folk remedy is strong hot chicken broth with lots of garlic and dandelion leaves.

Alcohol robs your body of essential vitamins, especially vitamin C and the B vitamins. If you don't feel like eating, at least take your multivitamin supplement.

❖ Hay Fever

Also known as allergic rhinitis, hay fever is an allergic reaction to pollen and other airborne substances such as house dust and mold. According to the National Institute of Allergy and Infectious Disease, hay fever affects some thirty-five million Americans, causing them to sneeze, sniffle, and have itchy, runny eyes.

Pollen from ragweed is one of the most common causes of hay fever, but pollen from many other plants can also be culprits. Some common plants include weeds such as sagebrush and lamb's quarters; trees such as oak, ash, hickory, elm, pecan, box elder, and mountain cedar; and grasses such as timothy, Bermuda, and Kentucky bluegrass. Despite its name, hay fever is rarely caused by hay; rose fever, an old-fashioned name for hay fever, is also misleading, because pollen from colorful or scented flowers rarely causes allergic reactions.

There is no cure for airborne allergies. Avoiding pollen, house dust, and mold will help reduce your hay fever symptoms, but these substances are often so prevalent that exposure is inevitable. Staying in an air-conditioned space can help, as can some kinds of air filters. Both reduce the amount of allergens in the air. Many doctors suggest over-the-counter or prescription antihistamines to help control the symptoms. Allergy shots (immunotherapy) can often help reduce the severity of allergic reactions. Don't try to desensitize yourself with bee pollen—a severe allergic reaction could occur.

Some hay fever sufferers claim that eating a cup or two a day of live-culture yogurt helps ward off their symptoms. Others say that eating lots of onions helps, perhaps because the antioxidant substance quercetin in the onions can help block the allergic response.

Some doctors suggest hay fever sufferers avoid foods that contain salicylates, such as berries, almonds, and apricots. These foods can trigger asthma attacks in sensitive individuals and may have an adverse affect on hay fever as well. (See the section on Asthma for more information.) Smoking, a smoky environment, and drinking alcohol can seriously aggravate your hay fever and should be avoided.

See also Allergies; Food Allergies.

❖ Headaches

Headaches are an extremely common ailment, affecting almost everyone sooner or later. In fact, according to the National Headache Foundation, forty-five million Americans have headaches bad enough to seek the help of a doctor.

There are several different types of headaches, and a variety of different causes. By far the most common type—about 90 percent of all headaches—is the tension headache, characterized by dull pain and a feeling of tightness around the scalp and neck. Most tension headaches are caused by stress, fatigue, or depression. Headaches can also be caused by hangovers, hunger, caffeine withdrawal, some foods and food additives, allergies, and sinus problems.

If your headache is severe and debilitating or causes nausea, vomiting, or blackouts, you may be experiencing a migraine. These very painful headaches are discussed separately in the section on Migraine.

Diet can play an important role in relieving headache pain and preventing headaches from happening. Tension headaches, for example, often get better if you start eating a generally more nutritious diet on a regular basis. Headaches from hangovers have an obvious cure: stop drinking. Hunger headaches usually start just before mealtime. They're caused by a combination of muscle tension and low blood sugar, and are far more likely to occur if you're dieting or if you skip meals. Here, too, the solution is obvious: good, nutritious meals on a regular basis. You won't get hunger headaches, and you'll feel better in general. Caffeine withdrawal headaches are very common. If you drink caffeinated beverages on a regular basis (more than two cups a day) and skip your usual three o'clock cup of coffee, for example, you may get a mild headache. The headache generally goes away when you ingest some caffeine. If you're trying to cut back on caffeine, taper off gradually to avoid withdrawal headaches.

Some foods and food additives cause headaches in sensitive people. Monosodium glutamate (MSG), a very common food additive, is a well-known headache trigger. MSG headaches are sometimes called Chinese restaurant headaches because the additive is often used in Oriental cooking. Today, most restaurants, Chinese or otherwise, either no longer use MSG or will leave it out at your request. If MSG gives you headaches, however, you'll also have to read all food labels carefully, since MSG is commonly used in a wide variety of prepared foods, such as frozen dinners and baked goods. It's also found in seasoned salts, meat tenderizers, and some brands of soy sauce. Sodium nitrite and sodium nitrate are common food additives that can cause headaches. These substances are very often added to prepared meats such as hot dogs, bacon, salami, bologna, and ham. The artificial sweetener aspartame (NutraSweet) can also cause headaches in some sensitive people.

Some foods are very definitely triggers for migraine attacks. If you tend to get headaches, even if they're not migraines, you might get fewer if you avoid the same foods. Stay away from alcohol (especially red wine), avocados, bananas, broad beans, caffeine, aged cheese, chicken livers, chocolate, citrus fruit, fava beans, figs, herring, lima beans, MSG, nitrates, nitrites, nuts, papayas, peanut butter, pizza, plums, raisins, snow peas, sourdough breads, sour cream, and strawberries. Many headache-prone people say that avoiding anything fermented, pickled, or marinated helps.

Headaches can be triggered by other foods as well. If you get frequent, nonmigraine headaches, try keeping a food diary for several weeks. If you notice that you usually get a headache within forty-eight hours of eating a particular food, that food could be a trigger for you. Avoid it.

Cluster headache is a relatively rare but very painful ailment. These headaches begin suddenly and unexpectedly; the pain is around or behind one eye. Attacks occur in clusters or groups for days, weeks, or even months at a time, and then may disappear completely for a year or more. Most cluster headache sufferers are men between the ages of twenty and thirty. There is some evidence that excessive alcohol use and/or smoking triggers cluster headaches.

For information on other types of headaches, see the sections on Food Allergies, Hay Fever, Premenstrual Syndrome (PMS), and Sinusitis.

❖ Hearing Problems

Two of the most commonly experienced hearing problems are sometimes related to what you eat: hearing loss and tinnitus (ringing in the hears).

A slow, progressive decline in hearing could be the result of a vitamin D deficiency that affects the cochlea, a snail-shaped bone in your inner ear. This is because vitamin D is essential for maintaining your bones, including the tiny bones in your middle and inner ears. If a vitamin D deficiency causes the cochlea to become porous, it will not transmit messages to the auditory nerve, resulting in hearing loss. A diet that is high in vitamin D can help restore some hearing if damage to the cochlea is causing the loss. The recommended dietary allowance for adults for vitamin D is 5 to 10 micrograms (200 to 400 IU). Fatty deep-sea fish such as salmon, canned sardines, mackerel, and herring are an excellent source of vitamin D; shrimp and fortified milk are good sources. However, too much vitamin D (more than four times the RDA) can be toxic.

Tinnitus is an irritating problem that usually affects older adults. It's often described as a ringing in the ears, but the sound can also be a buzz, pop, or hum. Prolonged exposure to high noise levels is one cause of tinnitus; people who work around jackhammers, jet engines, heavy machinery, and other noisy apparatus are more likely to develop it. According to the American Tinnitus Association, about fifty million Americans have tinnitus to some degree; of that number, twelve million have it severely enough to seek medical help. Tinnitus does not cause hearing loss, although most people who have hearing loss experience some tinnitus. More than 200 different prescription and nonprescription drugs list tinnitus as a potential side effect.

Alcohol, nicotine, caffeine, some prescription drugs, and aspirin all make tinnitus worse and should be avoided. Some foods naturally contain salicylates, the same substance found in aspirin. If you have tinnitus, you might want to avoid almonds, apples, apricots, most berries, cherries, grapes, nectarines, peaches, plums, prunes, and raisins. Some people with tinnitus find their symptoms are improved if they take supplemental vitamin A, zinc, and calcium. Avoid megadoses of vitamin A. Prolonged high doses are toxic to the liver.

❖ Heart Attack

About one and a half *million* Americans have heart attacks every year. The leading cause of death in the United States, heart attacks claim about 490,000 lives annually. A heart attack (also known as a myocardial infarction or coronary) occurs when one of the coronary arteries that supply blood to the heart is greatly narrowed or blocked. The blood supply to the heart is reduced or cut off; as a result, part of the heart muscle doesn't get the blood and oxygen it needs and begins to die.

High blood pressure, high blood cholesterol, cigarette smoking, and lack of physical activity are the major risk factors for heart attacks; other risk factors include obesity and diabetes. Having a family history of heart disease, being male, being African-American, and just getting older are additional risk factors.

Heredity, sex, race, or age are factors that are beyond your control, but you can certainly do something about the other risk factors. Quitting smoking, losing weight, getting more exercise, cutting back on alcohol, eating a low-fat, high-fiber diet, and taking steps to control your blood pressure and diabetes can sharply reduce your chances of having a heart attack. (See the sections on Angina, Atherosclerosis, Diabetes, High Blood Pressure, and High Cholesterol for more information.)

Since the mid-1980s, doctors have suggested that people at risk for heart attacks eat five ounces of fish twice a week to help their blood flow better, open arteries, prevent clotting, lower blood pressure, and raise HDL (good) cholesterol levels; some people also take supplemental fish oil capsules. But do the omega-3 fatty acids found in fish oil, especially from deep-sea fish, help prevent a heart attack? In 1995, the results of a large-scale study by the Harvard School of Public Health showed that eating more fish didn't lower the risk of heart attack for healthy men between the ages of forty and seventy-five.

Whether or not all that extra fish oil helps, today, almost all doctors recommend that heart patients eat a varied diet that is high in fiber, low in fat, and contains lots of fresh fruits and vegetables. Add an onion, plenty of garlic, and a handful of unsalted nuts daily to help prevent blood clots and keep your arteries open. About 30 percent of your calories should come from fat, but avoid animal fat. Instead, substitute monounsaturated fats such as olive oil or canola oil. Studies show that monounsaturated fats can actually help protect your arteries against damage.

Can a drink a day help prevent heart attacks? It's possible. If you regularly drink alcohol, having one or two drinks a day—but absolutely no more than that—may help increase your levels of HDL cholesterol and provide some antioxidants; it also helps you relax. Red wine contains anticoagulants. If you are taking medication for a heart condition or any other condition, or if you have angina, you should probably avoid alcohol altogether. Check with your doctor to be sure.

Heart Attack Warning Signs

A heart attack is a medical emergency that requires immediate medical help. Look for these warning signs:

- An uncomfortable feeling of pressure, fullness, squeezing, or pain in the center of the chest that lasts for more than a few minutes
- Pain that spreads or radiates to the shoulders, neck, or arm, especially down the left arm
- Chest discomfort along with light-headedness, shortness of breath, fainting, sweating, or nausea

❖ Heartburn

Heartburn is a burning feeling in the lower chest, usually along with a sour or bitter taste in the throat or mouth. (The taste gives heartburn one of its other names, sour stomach.) The pain of heartburn can be so severe that you may think you're having a heart attack, and sometimes people who are having a heart attack think it's just heartburn. Even so, heartburn has nothing to do with your heart—it's your esophagus, the ten-inch tube that leads from your mouth to your stomach, that's causing the trouble.

When you eat, food passes down the esophagus and into your stomach through a ringlike opening called the lower esophageal sphincter. The ring opens to allow the food in, then closes again to keep your acid digestive juices in the stomach where they belong. Sometimes, however, the ring doesn't close completely or doesn't stay closed. Food and stomach acid then back up (reflux) into the esophagus, causing the burning sensation of heartburn.

Occasional heartburn is very common. Eating too much or eating too quickly is one of the most likely causes, but many people have heartburn even when they don't overeat. Usually, something these people have eaten is causing the problem. Certain foods are well known to cause heartburn. Chocolate, spearmint, peppermint, onions, fatty or fried foods, and alcohol all relax the sphincter muscles and make reflux more likely. Other foods, such as juices, coffee, carbonated drinks such as soda pop and beer, and milk can increase the amount of acid your stomach produces and cause heartburn. Acidic foods such as tomato juice, tomatoes, citrus juice, coffee, and some spicy foods can irritate the esophagus; if you're already having heartburn, these foods will make the problem worse. Some people get heartburn from other foods. If you notice that something you eat consistently gives you heartburn, cut back on it or eliminate it from your diet. If you have chronic trouble with heartburn, a high-protein, low-fat diet may help.

Fortunately, some simple food remedies for heartburn are very effective. The simplest of all is to just slowly drink a glass of cold water. This can wash the acid back into your stomach and relieve the pain. Some people claim that the juice of a raw potato, mixed half and half with water, does wonders. Others say that drinking a tablespoon of apple cider vinegar mixed into 8 ounces of water during meals keeps them from getting heartburn. Over-the-counter antacids are often very helpful. If you need to avoid salt, however, stay away from the brands that contain sodium bicarbonate. If you are pregnant or have kidney problems, talk to your doctor before taking antacids.

There are some other practical steps you can take. Lose weight if you are too heavy. If you smoke, stop. Avoid tight-fitting clothing that puts pressure on your abdomen. Don't eat right before lying down—wait two to three hours. Many people find that elevating the head of the bed by about six inches helps relieve reflux problems. Heartburn can sometimes be a side effect of medications. If you think your medicine is causing heartburn, talk to your doctor or pharmacist.

Heartburn is sometimes a symptom of a more serious problem such as ulcers. If your heartburn is very severe, or if you have it more than three times a week for over two weeks, call your doctor. Also call your doctor if you have trouble swallowing or pain when you swallow, if you vomit blood, if your stools are bloody or black, if you're short of breath, dizzy, or light-headed, if the pain goes into your neck and shoulder, or if you break out into a sweat when you have the pain.

See also Hiatus Hernia: Ulcers.

❖ Hemorrhoids

Hemorrhoids are one of the most common ailments. Some twenty-five million Americans suffer from the pain, itching, and discomfort hemorrhoids cause. You can develop hemorrhoids when the special veins in the lower rectum at the junction of the anal canal become swollen and bulge out beneath the thin layer of tissue that covers them.

Internal hemorrhoids occur in the upper portion of the anal canal and may cause pain, burning, itching, or aching in the area. These hemorrhoids may also bleed, leaving bright red blood on the stool or on the toilet paper after a bowel movement. *External hemorrhoids* occur under the surface of the skin at the anal opening. They tend to disappear after a few days, but then they come back. External hemorrhoids produce pain, swelling, burning, and itching of the overlying skin.

What causes hemorrhoids? Anything that puts stress and pressure on the network of delicate hemorrhoidal veins in the rectum. A low-fiber, high-fat diet is the major culprit, because it leads to constipation or straining during bowel movements. Lack of exercise, sitting or standing for long periods, being overweight, or doing a lot of lifting can all contribute to hemorrhoids. Pregnant women often develop hemorrhoids because of the weight and pressure of the growing baby. These hemorrhoids usually go away after the baby is born.

In most cases, you can easily treat your hemorrhoid symptoms yourself. The pain and itching can be relieved with plain petroleum jelly, witch hazel, or a nonprescription cream. Sitz baths or warm compresses are also very helpful

The best treatment for hemorrhoids, however, is to avoid constipation and straining by eating a high-fiber diet. The fiber makes your stool softer and bulkier so that it passes much more easily. Add plenty of fresh fruits and vegetables to your diet, along with whole grain breads and cereals. Avoid low-fiber foods such as cheese, white bread, pastries, and meat. Some people find that particular foods, such as coffee or nuts, aggravate their hemorrhoids. If you notice that something you eat or drink makes your hemorrhoids worse, avoid those foods. Drink plenty of liquids—six to eight glasses a day—and get regular exercise.

If your hemorrhoids are very painful or bleeding a lot, call your doctor.

See also Fissure.

❖ Hepatitis

Hepatitis simply means inflammation of the liver. In most cases, hepatitis is caused by a virus; in some cases, it is caused by toxins such as drugs or alcohol. Because your liver performs many vital functions as your body's chemical factory, hepatitis is always cause for concern.

Five different kinds of viral hepatitis have been identified. In the United States, the most common form (more than half of all cases) is hepatitis A (sometimes called infectious hepatitis). The virus is excreted through the feces, so it is usually spread by poor hygiene. Epidemics of hepatitis A can be spread when food, water, or shellfish beds are contaminated. Hepatitis B (also called serum hepatitis) infects about 300,000 people in the United States every year. In this case, the virus is found in all the body fluids of the infected person. Hepatitis B is usually spread by intimate contact with an infected person, although it can also spread through contaminated instruments used for tattooing, body piercing, drug injection, and the like. The other forms of hepatitis—C, D, and E—are less common. Hepatitis C (also called non-A, non-B hepatitis) affects some 150,000 Americans every year. It is primarily spread through blood transfusions. Hepatitis D is a liver infection found only in conjunction with hepatitis B. Hepatitis E (sometimes called epidemic or waterborne hepatitis), is spread by contaminated water. So far, it is not a common illness in America, but epidemics have occurred in Mexico.

The symptoms of hepatitis vary a lot from person to person. Sometimes they are so mild that you're not really sick or think you just have an intestinal flu. The early signs are quite similar to flu: fatigue, joint and muscle pain, and loss of appetite. Later on, you may also be nauseous, vomit, have diarrhea, and run a low-grade fever. Your liver (the upper right side of your abdomen) may feel tender, and you may develop jaundice (yellow skin).

Hepatitis A and B usually clear up by themselves in about a month to six weeks, although it may take three or four months before you feel completely yourself again. The best treatment is rest and a good diet. Most doctors recommend a diet that is low in fat, dairy products, and sugar, high in complex carbohydrates and fresh fruits and vegetables, and has absolutely no alcohol. You should also avoid over-the-counter drugs such as acetaminophen (Tylenol) and ibuprofen (Advil), since these drugs could harm your liver. If you take other drugs, discuss them with your doctor.

The biggest problem for hepatitis patients is nausea and loss of appetite. Try eating frequent small meals instead of three large ones. Drink plenty of liquids. In addition, taking a daily multivitamin and getting some extra vitamin A and all the B vitamins can help your liver recover faster. Don't overdo, however too much vitamin A is actually toxic to your liver.

You can avoid hepatitis A by good hygiene, not drinking the water in contaminated areas, and not eating raw shellfish. There is an effective vaccine for hepatitis B. People who are at risk for the disease (health care workers, for example) should discuss the vaccine with their doctor.

Hepatitis A and B usually go away without any long-term effects; the other types are more likely to lead to serious complications and lifelong liver disease. If you think you have hepatitis, see your doctor at once.

❖ Herpes

Herpes is the name of a group of viruses. Herpes simplex type 1 (HSV-1) is the virus that causes cold sores (see the section on Cold Sores for more information). Herpes simplex type 2 (HSV-2) is the virus that causes genital herpes. Both forms of herpes simplex cause painful blisters and sores. Genital herpes is now a very common sexually transmitted disease. About 16 percent of all Americans between the age of fifteen and seventy-four have HSV-2—that's about thirty million people, or one in every six.

Genital herpes is easily spread by sexual contact. Symptoms usually develop within two days to three weeks. Usually, the first symptoms are redness and inflammation in the genital area; next, one or more blisters or bumps appear. The blisters quickly break and become painful open sores. The area is usually painful and may itch, burn, or tingle. Often you have flulike symptoms as well, with swollen glands, headache, muscle aches, or fever. During an active infection avoid intercourse. Even a latex condom may not protect your partner against catching herpes from you during this time. Although you may have no visible signs of herpes, you can still pass it on to your partner. If you have herpes, always use a condom.

A first attack of genital herpes can last for several weeks. Eventually, the area heals and the symptoms subside, but herpes never really goes away. Some people have only occasional, mild flare-ups, but many people have more frequent recurrences, often four or more times a year. Fortunately, recurrences are usually far less severe than the initial attack, and they generally get less severe with time.

Many people with genital herpes say that stress, illness, fatigue, being out in the sun, menstruation, or eating certain foods trigger their outbreaks. Some people claim that coffee, alcohol, sugary foods, colas, or yeast trigger recurrences. There's no real evidence one way or the other, but if you notice that a particular food seems to be related to recurrences, avoid it.

Many people have tried using dietary supplements of the amino acid lysine to control genital herpes attacks. Lysine is found in milk, yogurt, eggs, cheese, and meat. Scientific studies have produced mixed results, but some people feel that lysine supplements help them. Another amino acid, arginine, has been implicated in outbreaks in some people. Foods rich in arginine include chocolate, nuts, seeds, whole grains, corn, and beer. Again, the scientific evidence for this is slim, but avoiding arginine seems to work for some people. There is some evidence that eating a diet rich in vitamin A and iron could help reduce recurrences.

Most physicians feel that a nutritious, well-balanced diet is the best defense against herpes recurrences. Avoid alcohol, since drinking can reduce your nutritional status and depress your immune system. A daily multivitamin supplement is probably a good idea, but expensive megadose vitamin therapy is generally worthless against herpes. Megadoses of vitamin C or vitamin A could actually be harmful.

For more information about genital herpes, contact the National Herpes Hotline at 919/361-8488 or the Herpes Resource Center at 800/230-6039.

❖ Hiatus Hernia

In order to reach your stomach, your esophagus (the tube that leads from your mouth to your stomach) must pass through an opening—a hiatus—in your diaphragm. (Your diaphragm is a dome-shaped sheet of muscle that separates your abdomen from your chest and also helps you breathe.) The muscles around the hiatus can weaken and allow the abdominal part of the esophagus and sometimes part of the upper stomach to protrude up into your chest, a condition known as a hiatus hernia or a hiatal hernia. The most common symptom is severe heartburn when you lie down.

Hiatus hernia is quite common, particularly among overweight, older people. Many people with the condition have no symptoms. Some, however, experience acid reflux—better known as heartburn—when stomach acid is pushed up into the esophagus.

There are several self-help steps you can take to relieve hiatus hernia problems. If you are overweight, lose weight.

Because lying down lets stomach acid flow more easily into your esophagus, elevate the head of your bed by six inches or so (raise the bed itself—don't use pillows). Avoid tight clothing, stooping, or lying down immediately after eating. Many people find that eating several small meals a day instead of two or three large ones helps relieve their symptoms. Alcohol and tobacco usually worsen hiatus hernia symptoms. If you drink, cut back or stop. If you smoke, stop.

For more information on how to relieve the symptoms of acid reflux, see the section on Heartburn.

❖ High Blood Pressure

Blood vessels called arteries carry blood from your heart to the rest of your body. Blood pressure is the force of that blood as it pushes against the walls of the arteries. Every time your heart beats (about sixty to seventy times a minute when you are resting), it pumps blood out to the arteries. Your blood pressure is at its greatest when the heart contracts and pushes blood out. This is called systolic pressure. When the heart is at rest between beats, your blood pressure falls. This is called diastolic pressure. Blood pressure is always given as two numbers: the systolic and diastolic pressure. The measurement is written one above or before the other, with the systolic number on top or first.

Blood pressure is measured with an instrument called a sphygmomanometer. A cuff is wrapped around your upper arm and inflated to stop the blood flow in your artery for a few seconds. As air is released from the cuff, the sound of your blood rushing through the artery can be heard through a stethoscope. The first sound heard is the systolic blood pressure; the last sound is the diastolic pressure. At the same time, the changing pressure is registered on a gauge or mercury column.

Normal blood pressure ranges from below 130 to 140 systolic and below 85 to 90 diastolic. If your blood pressure is less than 140/90, then it is considered normal. High blood pressure, or hypertension, is anything above 140/90. High blood pressure is classified by stages; it gets more serious as the numbers get higher.

For most people, there is no single known cause of high blood pressure. When the cause is unknown, this type of high blood pressure is called *essential hypertension*. It can't be cured, but in most cases it can be controlled. And controlling hypertension is very important to your health: uncontrolled high blood pressure can lead to arteriosclerosis (hardening of the arteries), heart attack, enlarged heart, kidney damage, or stroke. High blood pressure itself generally has no symptoms or warning signs. The only way to know if you have it is to have your blood pressure checked regularly. If it is high, you can take steps to lower it. If your blood pressure is normal, you can learn how to keep it that way.

Anyone can develop high blood pressure. There are some important steps you can take, however, to help prevent the problem or help control it if you do develop hypertension:

- Maintain a healthy weight. Lose weight if you are too heavy.
- Be more physically active.
- Choose foods that are lower in salt and sodium.
- Choose foods that are lower in saturated fats.
- If you drink alcoholic beverages, drink in moderation—no more than two drinks a day.
- If you smoke, stop.

It's not clear why salt and sodium strongly affect the blood pressure of some people and not of others. If you have high blood pressure, it's best to be on the safe side. Try to limit your salt intake to 2,400 milligrams (about a teaspoon) a day. Substitute other seasonings, such as garlic, onion, lemon juice, and other spices, for the salt. Remember that salt is widely used in many prepared and processed foods. It is also a major ingredient in condiments such as steak sauce.

There is some evidence that certain dietary supplements can also help prevent high blood pressure. Eating foods rich in potassium appears to protect some people. Good dietary sources of potassium include apricots, bananas, dried beans and peas, fish, lean meats, milk, orange juice, peaches, potatoes, prunes and prune juice, spinach, sweet potatoes, and yogurt.

Population studies have shown that populations with low calcium intakes have high rates of high blood pressure. While it is unclear that taking calcium supplements will prevent high blood pressure, eating a diet rich in calcium-containing foods will help you get the Recommended Dietary Allowance of calcium. In general, adults need 800 to 1,000 milligrams a day of calcium; pregnant and nursing women need 1,200 milligrams a day. Milk and dairy products such as cheese and yogurt are high in calcium; low-fat and nonfat dairy products have even more calcium than the high-fat types. Other good dietary sources of calcium include dark green leafy vegetables such as kale and mustard greens, broccoli, cooked dried beans and peas, canned fish with the bones (sardines, for instance), and tofu (bean curd).

Magnesium is another mineral that may alter your blood pressure. Too little magnesium can make your blood pressure go up. Doctors caution against taking supplemental magnesium. Since the amounts you need are quite small, supplements could provide too much, which could cause additional problems, such as diarrhea. Supplemental magnesium could also interfere with other medications you may be taking. Instead, get your recommended dietary allowance of 300 to 350 milligrams a day by eating foods such as nuts, seeds, whole grains, dark green leafy vegetables, and cooked dried beans and peas.

Many researchers feel that a diet high in omega-3 fatty acid can help prevent or lower high blood pressure. Omega-3 fatty acid, also called fish oil, is found in deep-ocean fatty fish such as salmon, mackerel, anchovies, sardines, herring, and tuna. Today, many doctors recommend that patients with high blood pressure eat a small portion of fatty fish two or three times a week. It might also be a good idea to substitute olive oil for other oils in the diet. This monounsaturated fat seems to help lower blood pressure.

Several vegetables seem to have beneficial effects on high blood pressure, for reasons that are not clearly understood. Celery, for example, is a traditional remedy for high blood pressure. Eating a couple of stalks a day can be helpful. Garlic and onions contain adenosine, which relaxes the blood vessels and make then open up, lowering blood pressure. The fiber in all fruits and vegetables seems to have an overall beneficial effect on your blood pressure.

In general, lowering the amount of saturated fat in your diet will not have a direct effect on your blood pressure. However, a diet high in fresh fruits and vegetables and low in saturated fats is good for your heart; it can also help you lose weight or maintain your current weight, which will help control your blood pressure.

If you already have high blood pressure, your doctor may suggest that you avoid caffeine. If you don't have high blood pressure, however, there is no evidence that caffeine will cause or prevent hypertension.

See also Diabetes; Dialysis.

❖ High Cholesterol

Cholesterol is a waxy, fatty substance found in all parts of your body. Your body needs cholesterol to help make cell membranes, some hormones, and vitamin D. The cholesterol in your body comes from two sources: your body and your food. Blood cholesterol is made by your liver; in fact, your liver makes all the cholesterol you need. Dietary cholesterol comes from animal foods such as meat, poultry, eggs, fish, and milk and dairy products. (Plant foods have no cholesterol.) Eating too much dietary cholesterol can make your blood cholesterol level go up, and the higher your blood cholesterol level, the greater your chance of developing coronary heart disease. The reason for this is that the excess cholesterol in your blood builds up on the walls of the arteries that carry blood to your heart. Atherosclerosis, the term for this buildup of fatty plaque, narrows or even blocks the arteries that bring oxygen to the heart muscle. The eventual result is angina or a heart attack.

Lowering your blood cholesterol level slows the buildup of plaque; in some cases, it can even help reduce the buildup that is already there.

LDL vs. HDL

Just like oil and water, cholesterol and blood don't mix. In order for cholesterol to travel throughout your body in the blood, it is coated with a layer of protein to make a lipoprotein. There are several different kinds of lipoproteins, but the two most important are low-density lipoprotein (LDL) and high-density lipoprotein (HDL). Most of the cholesterol in your blood is carried as LDL cholesterol; only about a third to a quarter is carried as HDL cholesterol. But too much LDL cholesterol in the blood can lead to cholesterol buildup in the arteries. That's why LDL cholesterol is often called "bad" cholesterol. HDL cholesterol actually helps remove cholesterol from the blood and prevent the fatty buildup. That's why it is often called "good" cholesterol. In general, then, the goal is to lower your LDL (bad) level and raise your HDL (good) level.

A number of factors influence your blood cholesterol level. Age, sex, and heredity are all important factors. Blood cholesterol levels in both men and women begin to rise around age twenty. Women before menopause generally have levels that are lower than men of the same age. After menopause, however, a woman's LDL level goes up. If you have close relatives who have high levels of LDL cholesterol or a history of heart disease, your body is more likely to make a lot of LDL cholesterol and deposit it in the walls of your arteries.

You can't do much about your age, sex, or heredity, but you can do something about the other risk factors: your diet, your weight, and your activity level. What you eat has a big effect on your cholesterol level. If you eat a lot of saturated fats or dietary cholesterol, you can elevate your cholesterol levels. Consuming too many calories and becoming overweight can also raise your level of LDL cholesterol and lower your HDL level. On the other hand, increasing your physical activity can lower your LDL cholesterol level and raise your HDL level.

To measure your blood cholesterol levels, your doctor will take a blood sample and send it to a laboratory. The levels are measured in milligrams per deciliter, abbreviated as mg/dL. The charts below list the categories of cholesterol levels.

Blood Cholesterol Levels

Total Blood Cholesterol/HDL Cholesterol

Level	Category
35 mg/dL or less	low
36 to 199 mg/dL	desirable
200 to 239 mg/dL	borderline high
240 mg/dL	high

LDL Cholesterol

Level	Category
129 mg/dL or less	desirable
130 to 159 mg/dL	borderline high risk
160 mg/dL and above	high risk

Any cholesterol level of 200 mg/dL or more increases your risk of heart disease. A level of 240 mg/dL or greater is considered high cholesterol. If your cholesterol is at this level, you are more than twice as likely to develop heart disease as someone with desirable cholesterol. Unlike total cholesterol, where a lower number is better, the higher your HDL (good) cholesterol number, the better. If you do have high cholesterol, studies show that lowering it even a little can have a positive effect on your health. A healthy forty-year-old man with borderline high cholesterol (200 to 240 mg/dL) who lowers his cholesterol by just 10 percent can cut his risk of a heart attack by 50 percent. In other words, by making some simple changes in his diet, he can cut his chances of having a heart attack in half.

Eating to Lower Cholesterol

If your cholesterol levels are too high, your doctor will recommend that you eat foods low in saturated fat and dietary cholesterol, get more exercise, and lose weight if necessary. He or she may also recommend medication in some cases, but diet and exercise are the most important steps you can take.

The average daily intake of dietary cholesterol ranges from 220 to 260 milligrams for women and about 360 milligrams for men. These intakes are too high for most people. On average, Americans get 12 percent of their calories from saturated fat and 34 percent of their calories from total fat. The National Cholesterol Education Program recommends that you get less than 10 percent of your calories from saturated fat, 30 percent or less of your calories from total fat, and eat less than 300 milligrams a day of dietary cholesterol. If you follow these guidelines, also known as the Step I diet, your blood cholesterol levels will probably fall over the course of several months. If they don't, or if your cholesterol levels are very high to begin with, you might want to follow an even lower-fat diet, also known as the Step II diet. In this diet, less than 7 percent of your daily calories come from saturated fat, 30 percent or less of your daily calories come from total fat, and you eat less than 200 milligrams of dietary cholesterol in a day.

To lower your blood cholesterol, choose foods that are low in saturated fats, low in total fat, and low in dietary cholesterol. In general, lowering your intake of saturated fat is a lot more important than lowering your dietary cholesterol intake, but you should try to reduce both. (See A Closer Look at Fat on page 5 in the introduction for more information about fat and dietary cholesterol.) Choose foods that are high in complex carbohydrates and fiber. Maintain a healthy weight. If you are overweight, lose the extra pounds. Overweight adults with an apple shape—fat that collects in the abdomen—tend to have a higher risk for heart disease than those with a pear shape—fat that collects on the hips and thighs. One of the beneficial side effects of eating less fat and more whole grains, fruits, and vegetables is that you will probably also eat fewer calories and will lose weight.

Adding fiber, particularly soluble fiber, to your diet can help reduce your cholesterol level. In general, eating lots of fresh fruits and vegetables will have a beneficial effect. More specifically, cooked dried beans and peas are an excellent source of soluble fiber. Research suggests that just a cup of beans a day could significantly help to lower your LDL cholesterol level. Soybeans and other soy foods such as bean curd (tofu) and soy milk are particularly valuable, although soy sauce has no effect. Another excellent source of soluble fiber is oat bran, either by itself or as part of oatmeal. Just two ounces of oat bran a day (or one large bowl of oatmeal daily) can not only lower your LDL level, it can raise your HDL level. The process takes a few months, and while it may not work for everyone, it's certainly worth trying if your cholesterol levels are high. Other foods that are high in soluble fiber include apples, pears, and other fruits with a high pectin content, brussels sprouts, broccoli, carrots, turnips, and peas. Remember, plant foods have no dietary cholesterol.

Onions and garlic contain substances that apparently help reduce overall cholesterol and raise HDL levels. Raw onions and garlic seem to be the most effective. Some physicians now recommend half a raw onion or several raw garlic cloves (or garlic capsules) daily.

Avoiding eggs has become almost a phobia among people with high cholesterol. It is true that one egg yolk contains about 200 milligrams of dietary cholesterol and about 5 grams of fat, including 2 grams of saturated fat. (Egg whites have no fat or cholesterol.) On the other hand, eggs are a good source of protein, iron, and other nutrients. In addition, some studies indicate that eating eggs every day can actually raise the HDL levels of healthy adults. In the face of this confusion, most doctors still suggest you limit your intake to just four egg yolks a week. If you have low cholesterol and no other risk factors, you can probably safely eat more; if you have high cholesterol or other risk factors, however, limit your egg consumption to four a week or even less.

Saturated fats such as butter, lard, and animal fat, hydrogenated vegetable oils such as margarine and shortening, and tropical oils such as palm oil and coconut oil are all known to contribute to atherosclerosis and high cholesterol levels. Saturated fats are used in many prepared and processed foods, so read the labels carefully to avoid hidden fat. Also try to avoid the omega-6 fatty acids, which are found in polyunsaturated oils (sometimes called trans fats) such as corn oil, safflower oil, sunflower oil, and many vegetable shortenings. These oils oxidize easily and contribute to plaque buildup in your arteries. The American Heart Association recommends that you limit polyunsaturated fats to no more than 10 percent of your total daily calories.

Monounsaturated fats, such as olive oil, canola oil, and peanut oil, can actually be good for you. Olive oil contains antioxidant compounds that can help reduce oxidation of the LDL cholesterol in your blood. Similar compounds seem to be in the oils found in avocados and nuts such as walnuts and almonds. These foods aren't magic bullets, but the evidence suggests that substituting olive oil for other fats, or eating a handful of walnuts instead of cookies as a snack, could certainly help lower your cholesterol level.

Fish oil, otherwise known as omega-3 fatty acids, can also help improve your blood cholesterol by raising your HDL level. The best dietary sources of fish oil are fatty, deep-sea fish such as salmon, mackerel, herring, tuna, anchovies, and sardines. Eating just three ounces of fatty fish two or three times a week can have a beneficial effect.

Beta carotene, vitamin C, and vitamin E can help raise your HDL level. By eating more fresh fruits, vegetables, and whole grains, you will also be eating more of these essential vitamins.

Should you take supplements as well? Doctors are divided on the issue. Most would agree, however, that supplements in moderation probably won't hurt and could do a lot of good.

❖ Hives

Hives (urticaria) are small, very itchy, red, swollen bumps on the skin. Hives often appear in clusters; they tend to arise very suddenly and go away just as fast, often within an hour or two. Sometimes, however, hives can last for twenty-four hours or more. Generally, hives are annoying and itchy but not really dangerous. If you get hives in your mouth or throat, however, get medical help at once.

Often, hives are a reaction to something you have eaten or a medication you have taken. Foods that are likely to cause hives include shellfish, nuts, tomatoes, and berries, although other foods can cause hives in sensitive people. Medications that can cause hives include penicillin, sulfa, phenobarbital, anticonvulsants, and aspirin. Some people get hives as a reaction to stress. If a prescription medication gives you hives, stop taking it and call your doctor.

If you know that particular foods or medications cause you to get hives, avoid them.

❖ Hyperactivity

Hyperactive children have difficulty sitting still; they can be impulsive, inattentive, and easily distracted. In addition, they often have trouble tolerating frustration. Despite a lot of research in the area, the causes of hyperactivity are still basically unknown.

Many attempts have been made to treat hyperactivity through diet. Perhaps the best-known is the Feingold diet, named in 1973 for Dr. Benjamin Feingold. This diet eliminates all artificial flavorings, preservatives, and colorings and all foods containing salicylates (apples, berries, cherries, peaches, plums, tomatoes, and some other fruits and vegetables). Some parents claim their children show dramatic improvement on the Feingold diet, but it is unclear why. Controlled studies have never proven the diet to be effective; critics suggest that the extra attention the child receives is the real cause of the improvement.

Sugar is frequently blamed for hyperactivity in children, but again, this dietary approach has never been proven. In fact, some studies have shown the opposite: sugar can have a calming effect on children. Of course, too much sugar in a child's diet can cause appetite problems and tooth decay, so limiting the amount of sweets your child eats is generally a good idea.

Megadoses of vitamins are sometimes suggested for hyperactive children. Most doctors don't recommend this approach. It is unproven and can, in fact, cause diarrhea and other problems.

In desperation, some parents have resorted to drug treatment for their hyperactive child. Ritalin (methylphenidate) is one drug used to treat hyperactivity; amphetamines, specifically Dexedrine, is another. Long-term use of these drugs can cause serious nutritional problems for children because they tend to suppress the appetite. Children on these drugs eat less and don't grow or gain weight at a normal rate; their low appetites can also lead to vitamin and mineral deficiencies. A child being treated with these drugs should be under the care of a qualified pediatrician or psychiatrist.

❖ Hypoglycemia

The symptoms of hypoglycemia occur when you have too little glucose in your blood. When your body doesn't get the energy-providing glucose it needs, you can feel very hungry, tired, cold and clammy, dizzy, or nauseous. You might also tremble or get a headache. Sometimes your speech is slurred and people think you are drunk.

At one time, hypoglycemia was a popular diagnosis, but in fact, it is quite rare except among diabetics. If you have diabetes, you can become hypoglycemic easily, especially if you take too much insulin, skip or postpone meals, or exercise unexpectedly. To treat the symptoms, immediately eat something sugary such as a piece of candy or some sweet fruit juice. Your body needs the sugar, so don't have something that is artificially sweetened. It's important to know what your hypoglycemia symptoms usually are so that you can deal with them promptly. Delay can make the problem worse and even lead to a coma.

Some diabetics who have frequent episodes of hypo-glycemia find that taking supplemental chromium helps them control the problem. There's not much scientific re-search about the role of chromium in the diet. The daily recommended intake for adults is 50 to 200 micrograms, but some diabetics report that adding 200 micrograms daily helps control their hypoglycemia. Good dietary sources of chromium include brewer's yeast, orange juice, whole grain breads and cereals, molasses, cheese, and lean meats. Chromium supplements are also available. Niacin-bound chromium is believed to be more readily absorbed by your body than chromium picolinate. If you have diabetes, discuss adding chromium to your diet with your doctor before you try it.

If you're not diabetic, the effects of skipping meals or poor nutritional habits may show up as headaches, tiredness, irritability, and depression—symptoms that are sometimes vaguely attributed to low blood sugar. If you eat regular, nutritious meals that include lots of fruits, vegetables, and whole grains, and that are low in fat and processed foods, and if you avoid caffeine and alcohol, you will probably experience a miracle cure of your low blood sugar symptoms.

❖ Impotence

Impotence is the inability to achieve or maintain an erection long enough to have intercourse. Distressing as impotence can be, it is extremely common. Almost any man has experienced it every once in a while, often because of too much alcohol, drug abuse, stress, or exhaustion. Impotence for these reasons is almost always temporary and occasional. About ten to twenty million American men, however, are regularly impotent. Fortunately, in many cases impotence has a physical cause and can be helped.

Any disease that damages the delicate blood vessels of the penis can cause impotence. These include alcoholism, diabetes, atherosclerosis, kidney failure, Parkinson's disease, and stroke. Some medications (such as those for high blood pressure) can also cause impotence. Treating the underlying problem or changing medications often helps combat impotence.

Recent studies show that men who smoke cigarettes are 50 percent more likely to become impotent before the age of fifty. In addition, most of the other possible causes of impotence are made much worse if you smoke. More than half of all smokers with heart disease, for instance, are likely to experience impotence, compared to just 21 percent for nonsmokers with heart disease. If you smoke, stop.

A balanced, nutritious diet that is low in fat, and regular exercise can help keep your blood vessels in good condition, which in turn will help keep the blood flowing well to your genitals. Despite much myth, there are no foods that can cause or improve an erection. Because a zinc deficiency can cause a drop in the male hormone testosterone, some people believe that eating foods high in zinc (there are over 100 milligrams of zinc in six oysters) or taking zinc supplements can cure impotence. In fact, there's no evidence to support this.

❖ Incontinence

Urinary incontinence (loss of bladder control) is a condition that affects some twelve million Americans. It is a symptom, not a disease, and there's a lot you can do to keep it under control. Underlying causes of incontinence could be urinary tract or vaginal infections, certain medications, muscle weakness, enlarged prostate, nerve or muscle diseases or disorders, and some types of surgery. Don't be afraid to discuss incontinence with your doctor. He or she can help you identify the cause of the problem and find ways to treat it. Often, treating the underlying infection or prostate problem or changing your medication relieves the problem. Learning to do special bladder exercises to strengthen the muscles in the area can also help quite a bit.

If you drink a lot of liquids (more than six to eight glasses a day), this could be contributing to your incontinence. On the other hand, not drinking enough liquids could actually worsen the problem or lead to dehydration or a bladder infection. Do avoid alcohol, caffeine, and grapefruit juice—these are diuretics that make you urinate more. Cranberry juice, however, is generally beneficial to the bladder. If you have trouble with bladder infections, drinking cranberry juice on a regular basis may help (see the section on Urinary Tract Infections for more information).

❖ Infertility

If you decide to have a baby, it will take you on average about six months to a year to get pregnant. If you haven't conceived in that time, there is a chance that you or your partner is infertile. Infertility has many possible causes, so consult your doctor if you are having trouble conceiving. If there is a medical problem or abnormality, your physician can identify it and suggest treatments. Often, however, infertility has no apparent cause. In these cases, sometimes diet can make a difference.

Infertility in Women

A woman's weight can have an effect on her fertility. Weighing too little or too much affects your ability to conceive. Most doctors suggest that you try to lose or gain enough weight to be within 95 to 120 percent of your ideal weight. Of course, gain or lose weight while following a sensible diet.

Some evidence suggests that caffeine can have a negative effect on female fertility. If you drink more than a cup of coffee a day, try cutting back. Also avoid other sources of caffeine, including tea, cola, chocolate, and some soft drinks.

Cigarette smoking can have a negative impact on your fertility by altering your hormone levels. If you smoke, stop.

Eating well and getting sufficient vitamins and minerals is vitally important during pregnancy. If you are trying to conceive, start eating well now so that you and your baby will be getting good nutrition from the first moment of your pregnancy. (See the section on Pregnancy for more information.)

Infertility in Men

A common cause of infertility in men is a low sperm count. Alcohol, marijuana, and some drugs (both prescription and over-the-counter) can depress your sperm production. Culprits include some antibiotics and some ulcer medications such as Zantac and Tagamet. If you are taking a drug and your partner is having trouble conceiving, discuss the matter with your doctor. If a medication is depressing your sperm production, you might be able to switch to a different one.

Cigarette smoking can also depress your sperm count. If you smoke, stop.

❖ Inflammatory Bowel Disease

See Crohn's Disease; Irritable Bowel Syndrome; Ulcerative Colitis.

❖ Influenza

Influenza, or flu for short, is caused by a virus. Unlike colds, flu is most common in the winter and early spring, and it tends to occur in epidemics. Influenza is a more serious illness than a common cold, but the treatment is very much the same.

A case of the flu usually starts suddenly and makes you sick quickly. You may have a high fever, chills, muscle aches, sore throat, runny nose, headache, and a cough. You'll probably be sick for several days to a week, and it could take several weeks before you feel completely better.

Sadly, there is no cure for influenza. The best you can do is treat the symptoms. Stay home and rest, especially if you have a fever. Don't smoke; avoid secondhand smoke. Most importantly, drink plenty of fluids: six to eight glasses a day of water, fruit juice, chicken broth, uncarbonated soft drinks, tea, and the like. Don't drink alcohol, however.

Some people find that hot, spicy food helps clear their nasal passages, at least temporarily. Some people claim that eating garlic at the first hint of illness can ward off the flu; others say that garlic helps relieve flu symptoms and facilitates a quicker recovery. Cooked or raw garlic cloves are equally effective; if you don't like to eat the cloves, try garlic capsules instead.

More than a hundred different viruses can cause a cold, but only a few viruses cause influenza. For that reason, it's possible to make a flu vaccine. If you have heart or respiratory problems, are over age sixty-five, or have a chronic disease such as diabetes, ask your doctor about getting a flu shot.

See also Colds.

❖ Insomnia

About one-third of our lives is spent asleep, but getting a good night's sleep is a problem for about fifty million adult Americans. Insomnia, the most common sleep complaint, is the feeling that you have not slept well or long enough. Insomnia occurs in many different forms. Most often, it is characterized by difficulty falling asleep (taking more than thirty to forty-five minutes), awakening frequently during the night, or waking up early and being unable to get back to sleep.

Occasional insomnia can be triggered by many things: illness, anxiety, stress, minor ailments such as indigestion or a headache, some medications (prescription and over-the-counter), jet lag from travel, shift work, and so on. Long-term insomnia (lasting more than three weeks) can be a symptom of serious illness, chronic drug or alcohol abuse, too much caffeine, or depression.

Although insomnia can be a complex problem, some simple steps can help. Sleep experts agree that the best way to sleep better is to keep a regular sleeping schedule. Go to bed about the same time every night, but only if you are tired. Set your alarm to wake you at the same time every morning, even on weekends. If you have a poor night's sleep, get out of bed anyway. Lingering in bed or oversleeping will keep you from establishing a regular biological rhythm.

Alcohol (having a nightcap) may put you to sleep at first, but your sleep will probably be fragmented and you will probably wake up in the middle of the night when the alcohol wears off. If you can't sleep, don't have a drink. And if you drink in the evening less than two hours before going to sleep, that could be the cause of your insomnia. Smoking can also disrupt your sleep pattern because nicotine stimulates your nervous system. Try not to smoke in the evening. Better yet, don't smoke at all.

Caffeine is often the reason behind insomnia. If you're having trouble sleeping, avoid coffee, tea, cola, soda pop, and chocolate for at least six hours before bedtime.

Having a bedtime snack can help you get to sleep if you're hungry, but keep it light. Don't eat anything that could later cause heartburn and keep you up. A sugary or starchy snack such as crackers with cheese, toast with jelly, or a few cookies half an hour before bedtime helps many people get to sleep. A spoonful or two of honey might also work for you. Although there is no scientific evidence for it, many people swear by a glass of milk before bedtime. But don't drink too much before going to sleep—otherwise you might be awakened by the need to urinate.

Eating foods that are rich in the amino acid tryptophan may help relieve insomnia. This is because tryptophan is necessary for your body to make the neurotransmitter chemical called serotonin, which is one of the body chemicals that regulates sleep. Foods rich in tryptophan include milk, yogurt, cheese, tuna, turkey, bananas, peanut butter, and nuts. Eating these foods in combination with something starchy or sweet increases the effect of the tryptophan. Supplements containing tryptophan have been banned by the Food and Drug Administration.

Taken in small doses of 3 to 5 milligrams at bedtime, the hormone melatonin may be helpful for relieving insomnia from jet lag, night work, and other time-shifts. Supplements can be purchased in health food stores.

See also Jet Lag.

❖ Irritable Bowel Syndrome

The crampy pain, gassiness, bloating, and changes in bowel habits of irritable bowel syndrome have no known cause, yet they affect at least 10 to 15 percent of all American adults. Irritable bowel syndrome (IBS) is second only to the common cold as a cause of missed work.

In the past, IBS was often called colitis or spastic colon, but these terms are no longer used. (IBS should not be confused with ulcerative colitis, which is a more serious disease.) Sometimes irritable bowel syndrome can be severe and cause a great deal of distress and discomfort, but for many people it is a minor annoyance that can be largely controlled by diet, stress management, and medications prescribed by a physician when necessary.

If you have IBS, you may have diarrhea or constipation; many people with IBS experience periods of both. If you tend toward diarrhea, caffeine, fatty foods, and antacids containing magnesium may worsen the problem. If you tend toward constipation, try avoiding chocolate, milk, dairy products, and alcohol. In either case, many doctors suggest avoiding carbonated beverages and chewing gum to keep you from swallowing air that could aggravate your symptoms. Smoking can also worsen IBS symptoms.

Many people with IBS have symptoms following a meal. The larger the meal or the more fat it contains, the worse the symptoms may be. One way to keep meals from triggering IBS symptoms is to eat smaller portions or to eat smaller meals more often. Try to eat regular meals; eat slowly and chew your food thoroughly. Since fat often triggers IBS symptoms, eat a low-fat diet that is high in carbohydrates such as pasta, rice, whole grains, fruits, and vegetables. Milk and dairy products are triggers for many people; corn, wheat, the food additive monosodium glutamate (MSG), and the sweetener sorbitol are other common triggers. Avoid these foods and any others that you know aggravate your IBS symptoms. If you must avoid dairy products, be sure to get enough calcium by eating lots of leafy dark green vegetables; you should also discuss taking a calcium supplement with your doctor.

Dietary fiber can relieve the symptoms of irritable bowel syndrome quite a bit in many cases. Add high-fiber foods such as bran, whole grains, beans, fruits, and vegetables to your diet. Add over-the-counter fiber supplements only after discussing their use with your doctor. At first, you may experience bloating or gas, but as your system gets used to the additional fiber, this should diminish. Be sure to drink six to eight glasses of liquid every day as well—the fiber needs to absorb water to work.

See also Crohn's Disease; Ulcerative Colitis.

❖ Jet Lag

This modern ailment—unimaginable even fifty years ago—is caused by traveling rapidly through several time zones. Symptoms include insomnia, fatigue, disorientation, and digestive upsets. In short, jet lag sufferers complain that they feel like zombies.

Researchers have concluded that you need one day of adjustment for each time zone you pass through. If you travel west to California from New York, for example, you pass through three time zones (you gain three hours). In theory, you would be fully adjusted to the new time zone on the fourth day after your arrival. You probably don't want to wait that long to feel active and alert. Fortunately, there are some steps you can take to speed the adjustment period along.

One dietary approach that is often recommended is the feast-and-fast diet. This diet begins three days before your departure. On the first day, feast—eat as much as you want. On the second day, fast—eat lightly, but don't skip any meals. Feast again on day three. On the departure day, fast—eat light meals at their usual time. When you arrive, feast on whatever meal is appropriate for the local time. Many people who follow the feast-and-fast approach also cut back on caffeine during the four days before departure. Does this method work? There's no consistent proof, but many travelers claim it helps them adjust faster.

What you do during the flight will also have an effect on how you feel when you arrive. The air inside the plane is very dry, so to avoid dehydration drink plenty of liquids—except alcohol, which will dehydrate you even more. Eat the airline meals or snacks only if you are actually hungry. Bring along some fresh fruit, low-salt pretzels, or other low-fat foods for a healthy snack.

Once you land, most experts recommend that you get into the swing of things in the new time zone as quickly as possible. Eat normal meals at the normal times, and try to go to bed at your usual hour. Avoid napping during the day. It just slows up the adjustment process. If sleeplessness is a problem, try eating some tryptophan-rich foods such as bananas, cheese, milk, or turkey. The tryptophan acts as a natural sedative. Getting some exercise and being outdoors in the sunshine as much as possible will also help your internal body clock to adjust.

The hormone melatonin may be helpful for relieving jet lag symptoms, particularly insomnia. Your body clock is naturally regulated by melatonin, which is produced by your pineal gland. Taking small amounts of supplemental melatonin (about one milligram) at the right time and in the right amounts can help you reset your body clock more quickly when you have passed through a number of time zones. Melatonin supplements are available at health food stores. Use them with great caution, however. Too large a dose or a dose at the wrong time could lead to inappropriate or even dangerous sleepiness.

❖ Kidney Dialysis

See Dialysis.

❖ Kidney Stones

Kidney stones are, as the name suggests, pebblelike crystal deposits that form in the kidneys. Most kidney stones remain harmlessly where they are, but sometimes a stone passes from the kidney down through the ureter that leads to the bladder. This can cause the excruciating, spasmodic pain called renal colic—a condition that accounts for about one million hospitalizations every year, or more than 1 percent of the annual total.

Kidney stones are much more common among men than women, by a ratio of three to one. About 12 to 14 percent of all men experience at least one bout of kidney stone problems by the age of seventy. If you've had a kidney stone once, chances are good that you will have another one. Changing your diet, however, can help prevent a recurrence.

About 90 percent of all kidney stones are made of calcium oxalate. Because calcium is a waste product of meat digestion, many doctors recommend cutting back on animal protein. On the other hand, it's not a good idea to cut back sharply on your overall calcium intake. In fact, cutting back too far could lead to additional problems. Do, however, limit consumption of salt, sugar, alcohol, and caffeine since they all can increase the calcium levels in your urine. Magnesium-rich foods such as whole grains, bananas, potatoes, nuts, dark green leafy vegetables, seafoods, and cooked dried beans and peas may help block the formation of calcium stones.

Avoiding foods high in oxalate can also help prevent stone formation. Spinach, rhubarb, mustard greens, Swiss chard, and beet greens are very high in oxalate. Other high-oxalate foods include dandelion greens, baked beans in tomato sauce, okra, sweet potatoes, leeks, and peanuts. Most berries are high in oxalate, as are other fruits such as figs, oranges, grapefruit, grapes, plums, and prunes. Beverages such as beer, cocoa, colas, and tea contain high levels of oxalate; so do wheat germ, tofu, nuts, grits, and tomato soup.

Vitamin B_6 deficiency has been linked to oxalate kidney stones. If you've already had a kidney stone, discuss adding a vitamin B_6 supplement to your daily diet with your doctor. Megadoses of vitamin C over 2,000 milligrams a day have also been linked to kidney stone formation. If you have ever had a kidney stone, discuss any vitamin C therapy with your doctor before trying it.

Sometimes kidney stones are made up of uric acid, which is a waste product formed as the body breaks down purine, a substance found in foods containing protein. People who suffer from gout have an excess of uric acid and often develop this type of kidney stone. Doctors recommend cutting back on protein intake and avoiding foods that are high in purine, such as organ meats, herring, anchovies, sardines, beer, and wine if you have uric acid stones. Meats, seafood, fish, peas, beans, spinach, lentils, asparagus, and cauliflower, which are moderately high in purine, should be restricted to just one serving a day.

To help prevent either type of kidney stone from forming, it is important to drink a lot of fluids, which encourages a high level of urine production. Six to eight glasses a day of fluids is generally enough to produce a healthy 1 1/2 to 2 1/2 quarts of urine a day; drink more in hot weather or during times of heavy exertion.

❖ Lactose Intolerance

Lactose intolerance is the inability to digest significant amounts of lactose, the predominant sugar in milk and many milk products. The inability is caused by a shortage of the digestive enzyme lactase, which is normally produced by the cells that line the small intestine. Lactase breaks down the milk sugar into simpler forms that can then be absorbed into the bloodstream. When your body doesn't produce enough of the enzyme lactase to digest the dairy products you consume, the result can be diarrhea, gas, bloating, nausea, and cramps. The symptoms usually begin about thirty minutes to two hours after eating or drinking foods that contain lactose.

Between thirty and fifty million Americans are lactose intolerant. Certain ethnic and racial populations are more widely affected than others. As many as 75 percent of all African-Americans and Native Americans and 90 percent of Asian-Americans are lactose intolerant; many people of

Mediterranean descent are also lactose intolerant. The condition is least common among persons of northern European descent. (Lactose intolerance is not the same as an allergy to cow's milk.)

For most people, lactose intolerance is a condition that develops gradually over time. After about the age of two years, your body naturally begins to produce less lactase. If you are lactose intolerant, the symptoms will probably start to show up when you are in your late teens or early twenties, although often symptoms gradually develop in older people as their bodies stop producing lactase. People vary in their degree of lactose intolerance. Some may find that they can tolerate a small glass of milk but not a large one; others can eat ice cream but not drink milk. In addition, your level of lactose intolerance can change over time, usually for the worse.

Fortunately, treating the symptoms of lactose intolerance is simple: avoid milk and milk products in the quantities that make you ill. You can determine your optimal level largely through cautious trial and error.

If you are lactose intolerant, you can still get the calcium, protein, B vitamins, and other benefits of milk by drinking lactose-reduced milk, which is readily available in most supermarkets. Alternatively, you could purchase lactase tablets over the counter in a drugstore and add them to the milk yourself. Cultured buttermilk has slightly less lactose than an equivalent amount of regular milk. Some people find that they can digest chocolate milk but not plain milk. Also, many people find that they can better tolerate lactose if it is consumed as part of a meal. Take note: Neither raw milk nor acidophilus milk contains less lactose than regular milk. Raw milk isn't pasteurized, which could lead to illness.

After milk, ice cream is the biggest problem for most lactose intolerant people. The best approach is to simply avoid ice cream or eat it in small quantities after a regular meal. You could try chewing some lactase tablets before eating ice cream, but you will need to experiment to find the right dosage. Soft cheeses such as ricotta, cottage cheese, sour cream, farmer cheese, and the like can also cause problems. Most lactose intolerant people find that they can tolerate active culture yogurt and semisoft or hard cheeses such as Cheddar or Swiss.

People who are lactose intolerant need to watch out for the hidden lactose that is often added to prepared foods. Bread and other baked goods, processed breakfast cereals, instant potatoes, soups, breakfast drinks, powdered coffee creamer, whipped toppings, margarine, some lunch meats, salad dressings, and prepared mixes for pancakes, biscuits, and cookies often contain lactose, so read the labels carefully. When reading the list of ingredients, look for the words milk, lactose, whey, curds, milk by-products, dry milk solids, and nonfat dry milk powder. If any of these appear on the label, the product contains lactose.

Lactose is also used as the base for more than 20 percent of prescription drugs and about 6 percent of over-the-counter drugs. These products will be a problem only if you are severely lactose intolerant. If you are concerned, discuss the lactose content of the drug with your doctor or pharmacist.

If you can't drink milk, you may have trouble getting enough calcium in your diet. The recommended dietary allowance of calcium for an adult is 800 milligrams a day. Women who have not yet reached menopause and older women taking the hormone estrogen need at least 1,000 milligrams a day, roughly the calcium in a quart of milk. To get this much calcium without milk, try eating other milk products such as yogurt, processed cheese, and ice cream in quantities you can tolerate. Foods that are high in calcium but contain no lactose include broccoli, bok choy, kale, collard greens, turnip greens, salmon, sardines, tofu, and molasses.

❖ Leg Cramps

Many people have a good night's sleep rudely interrupted by painful muscle cramps in the calf or thigh. If these cramps occur often, the cause could be a calcium deficiency. Many doctors suggest a glass of milk before bedtime—an 8-ounce glass of 1 percent milk contains about 300 milligrams of calcium, or about a third of the Recommended Dietary Allowance. If you can't tolerate milk, try taking a calcium supplement tablet instead. Overall, make sure your daily diet contains enough calcium by eating a variety of calcium-rich foods, including broccoli, dark green leafy vegetables, sardines with bones, salmon, and such dairy products as cheese and yogurt.

Pregnant women sometimes experience leg cramps because of their changing calcium needs. If you're pregnant, your doctor will probably prescribe calcium supplements, which will also help relieve your leg cramps.

The quinine in tonic water can help prevent leg cramps. Try drinking 6 to 8 ounces an hour before bedtime. (If you wish, add some lemon juice to disguise the bitter taste.) You can also try stretching your legs in bed to help prevent cramps. Lie on your back and point your toes up and back toward your head; repeat a few times. If you get a leg cramp, stretching this way can help relieve it; standing up will usually also stop the cramp.

Taking diuretic drugs is another possible cause of leg cramps. Diuretics are often prescribed for high blood pressure and heart problems; over-the-counter diuretics are used by some women to relieve premenstrual water retention. If you take a prescription diuretic and have leg cramps, discuss the problem with your doctor. If you take a nonprescription diuretic and have leg cramps, stop using the product.

See also Restless Leg Syndrome.

❖ Liver Disease
See Alcoholism; Gallstones; Hepatitis.

❖ Lung Cancer

Today, lung cancer is the leading cause of cancer deaths among men, and it is nearing that level for women. In fact, about 59,000 American women die of lung cancer every year—more than die of breast cancer.

Without a doubt, cigarette smoking is by far the major cause of lung cancer. Smokers' chances of getting lung cancer are twenty to thirty times higher than nonsmokers. The more you smoke, the higher your risk. If you quit, however, your risk of lung cancer will begin to slowly decrease. Of course, it's best to never start and better to quit early, but you can benefit from giving up cigarettes even if you've already had lung cancer. Lung cancer patients who quit smoking are less likely to get a second cancer than are those who continue to smoke.

Some evidence shows that beta carotene (the precursor to vitamin A) and vitamin E may have a protective effect against squamous cell carcinoma (also called epidermoid carcinoma). This type of lung cancer is the most common type among men. It does not usually spread as quickly as other types of lung cancer. The evidence is far from conclusive, however. If you do smoke, taking megadoses of vitamin A and vitamin E will almost certainly have no protective effect and could be dangerous. The best way to prevent lung cancer is clear. Don't smoke.

See also Chemotherapy; Radiation Therapy.

❖ Lupus Erythematosus

Lupus erythematosus is a chronic autoimmune disease that causes inflammation of various parts of the body, especially the skin, joints, blood vessels, and kidneys. It has no known cause. For most people, lupus is a mild disease affecting only a few organs. For others, the disease is more severe and even life threatening. Between 1.4 and 2 million Americans have been diagnosed with lupus—more than have AIDS, cerebral palsy, multiple sclerosis, sickle cell anemia, and cystic fibrosis combined. Lupus affects 1 out of every 185 Americans; it occurs ten to fifteen times more often among women than men.

One type of lupus, called discoid lupus, is limited only to the skin. Patients get a red rash on the face, neck, and scalp. Systemic lupus is usually more severe than discoid lupus and can affect almost any organ or system of the body. The most common symptoms include achy or swollen joints, fever, prolonged fatigue, skin rashes, anemia, kidney problems, pleurisy, and sensitivity to sunlight.

Drugs such as aspirin, corticosteroids, and antimalarial medications often help control lupus symptoms. Although research is still in the early stages, there is some evidence that diet can also play a role. Many lupus patients have reported flare-ups of symptoms after eating particular foods. Research suggests that several common dietary plants, including soybeans, corn, spinach, and carrots, contain a plant protein that could trigger autoimmune antibodies in lupus patients.

In another study, a volunteer who ate alfalfa as part of a cholesterol-lowering study developed lupus symptoms. The effect was later duplicated in studies with monkeys. The amino acid L-canavanine was identified as the culprit. As a result, lupus patients are advised to avoid alfalfa sprouts and any health food products that contain alfalfa.

The omega-3 fatty acids found in fish oils seem to show promise as a way to help control lupus symptoms. Studies have shown that high doses of omega-3 in the form of capsules can help reduce lupus joint inflammation, although no more than aspirin does, and at a much higher cost. Most doctors suggest that lupus patients continue to take their usual medicines and simply add more fatty fish such as mackerel, salmon, herring, tuna, swordfish, cod, and halibut to their diet.

Many lupus patients report that their symptoms of sun sensitivity and inflamed skin are reduced when they take vitamin E in doses of 800 to 2,000 IU daily. If you have lupus, discuss taking supplemental vitamin E with your doctor before trying it.

❖ Macular Degeneration

Age-related macular degeneration is a blinding eye disease that affects the small area in the back of the eye called the macula. The macula is the central, most sensitive part of the retina. Macular degeneration destroys the sharp vision needed for seeing objects clearly, which can impair common daily activities such as driving and reading. Fortunately, macular degeneration almost never results in complete blindness, since peripheral vision is usually not affected.

The greatest risk factor for macular degeneration is simply age. The problem is rare among people under the age of sixty. Among people age seventy-five and older, the risk of macular degeneration is 30 percent. If you have high blood pressure, diabetes, or cardiovascular disease, you are more likely to develop macular degeneration. Women get macular degeneration more often than men. If you are white, you are much more likely to have macular degeneration than if you are African-American. Smoking may also increase your risk.

Sadly, there is little that can be done to help macular degeneration, although laser surgery can be useful in some cases. Prevention may be the best approach. Recent research indicates that people who eat foods high in carotenoids (the orange or yellow pigments found naturally in foods such as carrots) have a 43 percent lower risk of developing macular degeneration. Two carotenoids, lutein and zeaxanthin, have been shown to be particularly effective. Good dietary sources of these substances are dark green leafy vegetables such as spinach and collard greens. It's possible that the carotenoids are similar to natural yellowish pigments that are lost from the retina when macular degeneration occurs. Taking supplemental vitamin A, vitamin E, and vitamin C seems to have no effect on reducing the risk of macular degeneration, although they may be helpful for preserving your overall vision and in preventing cataracts.

See also Cataracts; Glaucoma.

❖ Menopause

As a woman reaches middle age, her reproductive life naturally comes to an end as her menstrual cycles gradually cease. Menopause (from the Greek words *menos,* meaning month, and *pauein,* meaning to cease) is characterized by a decline in the function of the ovaries, which in turn leads to decreased production of female hormones. Menopause generally occurs between the ages of forty and fifty-five; the average age is fifty-one. A woman is officially in menopause when she has not had a menstrual period for a year.

As your ovaries stop making the female hormones estrogen and progesterone, you are likely to experience some physical and emotional changes. Every woman experiences menopause differently. Some women feel very few effects of estrogen loss, while others feel the loss severely. A combination of modern medicine, dietary measures, and a positive outlook can make the transition far less troubling.

Hot Flashes

Probably the most common symptom of menopause is the hot flash. Over 75 percent of all menopausal women get them. Hot flashes are often described as a sudden wave of heat, causing flushing on the face and neck. The flashes can last anywhere from a few seconds to an hour, although most last just a minute or two. Unfortunately, they often occur at night and disrupt your sleep, leading to insomnia and fatigue. Many women have several hot flashes a day, while a lucky few have them only occasionally. Most menopausal women have hot flashes for a year or even two, but they almost always cease within five years. Although scientists still don't know exactly why hot flashes occur, they do know that estrogen supplements are very helpful for reducing or eliminating them. Many women find that alcohol, hot liquids, and spicy foods can trigger a hot flash. If this happens to you, avoid alcoholic beverages, choose cool or iced drinks, and cut back on the hot spices.

Vaginal Dryness

Because estrogen levels drop during menopause, the lining of the vagina becomes thinner, drier, and less elastic. These changes can cause discomfort during intercourse and can also lead to vaginal infections. Estrogen replacement therapy can be helpful for relieving vaginal dryness. Water-based vaginal lubricants, sold over the counter in any drugstore, are very effective. Avoid oil-based lubricants, since these can lead to infection.

Osteoporosis

A serious consequence of menopause can be osteoporosis, or thin, brittle bones caused by a loss of bone mass. After the age of about thirty-five, women begin to lose more bone than their bodies produce. For about six to eight years after menopause, the decrease in bone mass occurs faster. The result can be bones that break easily, which may cause crippling injuries that can lead to death.

To prevent osteoporosis later, you need to consume a lot of calcium now. Most doctors now recommend 1,000 to 1,200 milligrams of calcium daily for younger women and 1,500 milligrams a day for postmenopausal women. Milk and dairy products are an excellent source of calcium. One 8-ounce glass of nonfat milk contains about 300 milligrams of calcium; a cup of yogurt contains about 400 milligrams. Other good sources of dietary calcium include broccoli, dark green leafy vegetables, tofu (bean curd), sardines and canned salmon (with the bones), and cooked dried beans and peas.

Many women find it difficult to get enough calcium through their diet, especially if they are lactose intolerant and can't drink milk. Discuss your calcium needs with your doctor—supplemental calcium may be needed.

Tobacco, alcohol, and caffeine can interfere with your body's absorption of calcium. If you smoke, stop. Cut back on alcohol and caffeine.

To use calcium properly, you also need adequate levels of vitamin D. Your body produces its own vitamin D from exposure to sunlight and also gets it from your diet. As you age, however, your body's ability to make its own vitamin D is reduced, so it's especially important for menopausal women to get the recommended 400 IU a day. Good dietary sources of vitamin D are cod liver oil, fortified milk, egg yolks, tuna, salmon, canned sardines, shrimp, and liver. Bear in mind that most dairy products are not made with fortified milk and are not good sources of vitamin D. You can also take supplemental vitamin D, but this can be toxic at high levels. Discuss supplements with your doctor before you use them.

Weight-bearing exercise, such as walking, jogging, and bike riding, is also very helpful for building bone strength and preventing osteoporosis.

In addition to making sure you get enough calcium, vitamin D, and exercise, discuss estrogen replacement therapy with your doctor. Recent studies have proven that women who begin taking estrogen within five years of menopause and continue it for the rest of their lives have a substantially lower risk of bone fractures, and heart disease.

Diet and Menopause

Women who eat a low-fat or vegetarian diet report that they have fewer menopausal symptoms and that the symptoms they do have are less severe. Women who regularly eat soy products such as tofu and soy milk also report fewer and less severe symptoms. This is probably because soybeans contain large amounts of phytoestrogens, plant estrogens that are similar to human estrogen. Phytoestrogens are found at lower concentrations in other plant foods such as cabbage, garlic, oats, pineapple, peanuts, sesame seeds, and flax seeds.

The mineral boron may have an effect on estrogen levels. Although boron is found in many tissues in the body, no recommended dietary allowance has been established, and there are no known deficiency symptoms. One study, however, suggests that postmenopausal women who eat foods high in boron can naturally increase the level of estrogen in their blood. Foods that contain high levels of boron include most fruits, legumes such as soybeans and peanuts, and nuts such as almonds.

See also Osteoporosis; Urinary Tract Infections.

❖ Menstrual Cramps

During menstruation, the lining of a woman's uterus produces substances called prostaglandins, which help the uterus contract and expel its lining. Those same contractions, however, also produce the discomfort of menstrual cramps.

There are some useful dietary measures that can help reduce menstrual cramping. First, be sure you are getting enough calcium in your diet. Calcium helps regulate muscle tone; too little can lead to cramps. The recommended dietary allowance of calcium for women is 1,000 to 1,200 milligrams a day; postmenopausal women need 1,500 milligrams a day. The best dietary source for calcium is milk. One 8-ounce serving of nonfat milk has about 300 milligrams. Other good dietary sources for calcium include broccoli, dark green leafy vegetables such as spinach and kale, canned sardines and salmon (with the bones), and cooked dried beans and peas. If you find it difficult to get enough dietary calcium, consider taking supplements, particularly in the days just before and during your period.

Another mineral that plays a role in menstrual cramps is magnesium. This mineral has functions similar to calcium in the body. You need adequate amounts to help your body utilize calcium properly and help decrease menstrual cramps. The recommended daily allowance of magnesium for a woman is about 300 milligrams. Good sources of magnesium include nuts, cooked dried beans and peas, whole grains, soybeans, dark green leafy vegetables, and seafood. Other good sources are milk, bananas, avocados, wheat germ, and brewer's yeast. Be sure to eat some of these foods, along with calcium-rich foods, in the days just before and during your period.

If you normally have heavy menstrual flows, try eating a cup or so of pineapple every day for a few days just before and during your period. The manganese in the pineapple reduces the flow and helps relieve cramping. If your periods become unusually heavy or last longer than usual, however, see your doctor.

See also Premenstrual Syndrome (PMS).

❖ Migraine

A migraine is a severe headache, usually attacking just one side of the head, accompanied by a range of other unpleasant symptoms such as nausea, vomiting, aversion to light, and cold hands and feet. Migraines are a fairly common type of headache—some sixteen to eighteen million Americans, 70 percent of them women, get them.

Most migraines last for about six hours, although in some cases they can go on for longer. Many migraine sufferers experience warning signs, called the prodrome or aura, an hour or two before the headache strikes. The warning signs are usually visual, such as seeing flashing lights or zigzag patterns. Only about 20 to 30 percent of all migraine headaches begin with an aura, however.

The cause of a migraine is complex and not fully understood. Researchers believe that your levels of a substance called serotonin, which your body produces to help regulate the diameter of blood vessels, play an important role. If your serotonin levels fluctuate as a result of stress, low blood sugar, or changes in your estrogen level, a migraine could result. In addition, foods, especially those that naturally contain a substance called amine, can trigger a migraine. This is because amines affect the diameter of blood vessels; if your blood vessels open up (dilate) too widely, a migraine headache could ensue.

Amines of various sorts are found in many foods. Tyramine, for example, is found in aged cheeses, herring, organ meats, many nuts and seeds, peanuts, sauerkraut, and alcohol; octopamine is found in citrus fruits, and phenylethylamine is found in chocolate. Other foods that contain amines include most beans and legumes (pinto beans and lentils, for example) and fruits such as figs, dates, raisins, passion fruit, pineapple, papayas, avocados, red plums, and bananas. Aged, pickled, preserved, fermented, cured, or cultured foods can also be migraine triggers. If you get migraines, try avoiding alcoholic beverages, including beer and wine; sausage such as salami and pepperoni; cultured dairy products, such as sour cream and buttermilk; breads and cakes containing yeast; olives; and pickles.

Nitrites and nitrates, chemicals that are often added to processed foods, can also trigger migraine headaches. Processed meats such as sausage, ham, bacon, luncheon meats, and hot dogs often contain nitrites and nitrates. Monosodium glutamate (MSG) can be a migraine trigger for some people. MSG is often added to processed foods and soups and is also found in soy sauce, meat tenderizers, and seasoned salts. The caffeine in coffee, tea, or soft drinks may also be a factor in migraines. Most doctors recommend that migraine sufferers limit their caffeine intake to no more than two cups a day.

Of course, there is no guarantee that eliminating the above foods will keep you from getting a migraine, but there is good chance that some of them are triggers for you. If you get migraines often, discuss keeping a food diary with your doctor. By keeping a record of what you eat and how it affects your migraines, you can discover your own food triggers. You may find, for example, that you can eat citrus fruits in moderation (half a cup a day, perhaps), but that more causes a migraine.

In addition to avoiding food triggers, doctors suggest that migraine sufferers eat nutritious meals on a regular basis; five small meals a day may be preferable to three larger meals. Avoid skipping meals or fasting. Also avoid eating large amounts of carbohydrates, fats, protein, or sugar at one sitting.

See also Headaches.

❖ Mitral Valve Prolapse

The valves in your heart maintain the flow of blood in one direction and keep your circulation moving properly. The mitral valve controls the flow of blood from your left atrium into your left ventricle; from there, the blood goes out through the aortic artery to the rest of your body. In most people, the two flaps that make up the mitral valve are just the right size to close together tightly when your heart contracts. In some people, however, the flaps of the mitral valve are a bit too big or don't fit together exactly, so when the flaps come together, they either fail to close completely or balloon outward slightly. This condition is called mitral valve prolapse, and it's surprisingly common. By some estimates, anywhere from one out of every ten to one out of every twenty people has it; others estimate that about 5 percent of the population has it. About two-thirds of the people with mitral valve prolapse are women. You might learn that you have the condition only when a doctor listens to your heart through a stethoscope and hears the clicking sound the flaps make.

In almost all cases, mitral valve prolapse is completely harmless and has no symptoms. In some cases, however, mitral valve prolapse can cause symptoms such as shortness of breath, dizziness, palpitations, and racing heart. With rare exceptions, the symptoms are mild and go away in a few minutes on their own. In those few cases where mitral valve prolapse causes serious symptoms, treatment with beta-blockers or other drugs can be helpful. Because the symptoms can resemble those of anxiety or a panic attack, however, people with mitral valve prolapse are occasionally incorrectly diagnosed as having psychological problems.

Some patients find that reducing their caffeine intake can help prevent or lessen their minor mitral valve prolapse symptoms. Smokers who have mitral valve prolapse should make every effort to quit.

If you have mitral valve prolapse, discuss taking prophylactic antibiotics before any dental or surgical procedures with your doctor. The antibiotics keep bacteria from entering the bloodstream and infecting the valve.

See also Cardiac Arrhythmias.

❖ Morning Sickness

During the first three months of pregnancy, almost all women have some morning sickness—nausea and vomiting—but some unfortunate women have it for all nine months.

Although researchers still don't know exactly why morning sickness happens, there are some useful steps you can take to relieve the symptoms without drugs. Many women find that eating plain, unsalted crackers the moment they awaken in the morning—even before getting out of bed—can help quite a bit. Others find that eating small, frequent meals throughout the day instead of three larger meals is helpful. In general, avoid spicy, greasy, and strong-smelling foods; substitute easy-to-digest carbohydrates, such as rice or pasta, for meat if the taste or smell of meat makes you ill.

If you are vomiting a lot, it is very important to replace the fluid you lose. Avoid coffee and other caffeine-containing beverages and carbonated drinks; instead, try to drink water, broth, or fruit juice. Do not consume any alcoholic beverages during pregnancy.

See also Pregnancy.

❖ Motion Sickness

Car sickness, seasickness, and airsickness are all variations on the basic theme of motion sickness, or nausea and vomiting as a result of constant, unpredictable movement. Motion sickness is quite common. Even experienced sailors can get seasick on a rough day, so you shouldn't be surprised to find yourself hanging over the rail, too.

In some circumstances, motion sickness may be nearly inevitable, but there are some steps you can take to reduce or eliminate the symptoms. First, avoid fatty, greasy foods and those with strong odors. Eat a small, simple meal before the trip begins. If you must eat while traveling, stick to simple carbohydrates such as plain crackers, rolls, potatoes, and rice; fruits such as apples and bananas are usually easy to keep down. Avoid caffeine, carbonated beverages, and any sort of alcoholic beverage; stick to plain water.

A number of folk remedies exist for motion sickness. You could try sucking on a slice of lemon, eating some olives, or eating candied ginger. Eating plain, unsalted crackers or dry toast might also help.

To reduce the chances of motion sickness, try to avoid strong smells such as diesel fumes. Get plenty of fresh air, either by staying on deck, opening the car window, or aiming the air vent in your direction. If possible, position yourself so that you are looking straight ahead—it may help to sit in the front seat of the car, for example. If you know you get motion sickness and are planning to go on a cruise, discuss using a motion sickness patch with your doctor. The patch is placed on your skin and releases a continual flow of a motion sickness preventing drug into your bloodstream.

❖ Mouth Sores

Mouth sores, also called oral ulcers or canker sores, are a painful nuisance for many people. Recurrent mouth sores, known medically as aphthous stomatitis, afflict about 20 percent of the population. The sores are usually found on the tongue or the inside linings of the lips and cheeks.

The cause of mouth sores is not well understood. The sores don't seem to be caused by a virus or bacteria, and they're not contagious. In some cases, they may be the result of an allergic reaction to certain foods. Another cause may be the hormonal changes of the menstrual cycle in some women. In still other cases, mouth sores may be due to a nutritional deficiency, particularly of vitamin B_{12}, folic acid, or iron.

While your mouth sore is healing, avoid abrasive foods such as potato chips, which can stick in the cheek or gum and aggravate the sores. Similarly, avoid acidic and spicy foods.

If you notice that you consistently develop mouth sores within twenty-four hours of eating a particular food, you might be having an allergic reaction; try to avoid the problem food. If you think your mouth sores are related to a nutritional deficiency, try improving your diet. The recommended dietary allowance for vitamin B_{12} is very small—only 2 micrograms daily—but this nutrient is found only in animal foods, such as poultry, meat, and eggs, and in fermented foods. If you are a vegetarian, try adding a fermented soybean food such as miso to your diet. Folic acid is found in brewer's yeast, dark green leafy vegetables, broccoli, orange juice, beets, beef liver, and wheat germ. The recommended dietary allowance is 200 micrograms; however, pregnant women should try to get at least 400 micrograms daily. Good dietary sources of iron include organ meats, lean red meats, dried fruits such as raisins and prunes, whole grain breads and cereals, broccoli, strawberries, tomato juice, molasses, cooked dried beans and peas, and brussels sprouts. For folic acid, however, the recommended dietary allowance of 10 to 12 milligrams a day is hard to get solely through diet. If you think you're not getting enough iron, talk to your doctor about taking iron supplements.

❖ Multiple Sclerosis

Multiple sclerosis (MS) is a chronic disease of the central nervous system that causes varying degrees of interference with speech, walking, and other basic functions. MS symptoms can run the gamut from slight blurring of vision to complete paralysis, but the majority of people with MS do not become severely disabled and continue to lead productive and satisfying lives. About 350,000 Americans have MS, with nearly 200 new cases diagnosed every week. Multiple sclerosis often strikes people in their prime, most commonly between the ages of twenty and forty. Nearly twice as many women as men have MS. The cause is still unknown.

The symptoms of MS are caused by inflammation and scarring of tissue in the brain and spinal cord. This occurs because the disease destroys the fatty sheath that forms a covering for the nerve fibers of the central nervous system. Without the sheath, the impulses that travel along the nerves are disrupted, much as removing the insulation from around an electrical wire causes interference with the transmission of signals.

The symptoms of MS vary greatly, depending upon where the nerve damage occurs. Typically, someone with multiple sclerosis has periods of active disease, called exacerbations, and symptom-free periods, called remissions. One common feature of MS is that many symptoms worsen when patients are exposed to heat.

As of now, there is no cure for multiple sclerosis. Physicians can only treat the symptoms. In addition to medication, MS patients can often benefit from careful attention to diet. Although there is no evidence that a particular diet or nutritional supplement can help treat the disease, some of the symptoms of MS, such as bladder problems and constipation, can be helped by good nutrition.

Bladder problems affect almost everyone with MS at some point. To avoid urinary tract infections, MS patients need to drink lots of fluids in order to keep the bladder flushed. Many doctors recommend one or two glasses of cranberry, prune, apple, or apricot juice daily, along with four to six glasses of plain water. Avoid citrus juices, but take 1,000 milligrams of vitamin C four times daily to keep the urine acidified. This creates an unfriendly environment for bacteria. Avoid beverages containing caffeine.

To avoid constipation, MS patients need to add lots of fresh fruits, fresh vegetables, and whole grains to their diet; adding bran may also help. Again, drinking lots of fluids will help—six to eight glasses a day.

People with advanced MS may have difficulty chewing and swallowing. Your doctor can help you learn techniques that make swallowing easier. He or she can also refer you to a nutritionist who can teach you ways to change the form of your food to make it easier to eat and nutritionally sound. Thicker drinks such as milk shakes, juices in gelatin form, sherbets, and puddings are all good ways to increase fluids and nutrition. Foods that crumble easily, such as crackers, toast, and chips, should be avoided because they can cause choking. Soft foods that need less chewing, such as baked potatoes and stewed fruits, are good choices.

MS can cause severe fatigue. To keep up your energy levels, be sure to eat a good breakfast. It may also help to eat several small meals throughout the day instead of three larger meals, especially if you have trouble chewing and swallowing. If you're just too exhausted to make yourself something to eat, order in or keep some frozen dinners on hand for quick reheating in the microwave.

In general, the best overall diet for MS patients is a normal one based on the food pyramid. Numerous special diets that claim to miraculously cure or help multiple sclerosis have been tried. Although some seem to help a few people, at least for a time, none has been found to have genuine therapeutic value. Special diets may seem to work largely because MS is an episodic disease. Remissions attributed to diet may have simply occurred naturally. Neither the Swank diet nor the MacDougal diet has been accepted by the National MS Society's Medical Advisory Board as being effective, but these diets are not harmful. The Swank diet, for example, is basically just an extremely low-fat diet, while the MacDougal diet combines a low-fat approach with a gluten-free diet and supplemental vitamins and minerals. Beware of other diets that claim to be therapeutic; some are based on unproven theories that have never been tested in controlled studies. The same is true of therapies based on megadoses of vitamins or minerals. For example, injections of vitamin B_{12} will not benefit MS patients, because there is no evidence that the disease is caused by a vitamin B_{12} deficiency. Treatment with massive doses of vitamin C (sometimes called megascorbic therapy or orthomolecular therapy) is not only ineffective and possibly dangerous, it is also very expensive.

❖ Nail Health

The nails of your fingers and toes protect those sensitive digits from injury and infection. Like your hair, your nails are made of dead, hardened protein called keratin that is actually quite similar to the surface layer of your skin. Nail problems are usually not especially dangerous, but they can be painful and unsightly.

Deformed or discolored nails are usually the result of illness or injury, but sometimes they are caused by vitamin deficiencies. For example, iron-deficiency anemia can make your fingernails spoon-shaped, while a lack of calcium can cause dry, brittle fingernails. Overall, most dermatologists recommend a well-balanced, nutritious diet along with a daily multivitamin supplement for good nail health.

If you're still having nail problems a few months after improving your diet, try adding additional vitamin E (200 IU daily) and fish oil (1,000 milligrams daily). You could also try adding the nutrient biotin to your diet. Liver, oatmeal, brewer's yeast, egg yolks, soybeans, and bananas are excellent dietary sources of this B-complex vitamin; other good sources are cauliflower and legumes such as peas, peanuts, beans, and lentils. Don't bother drinking a glass of unflavored gelatin mixed with water. This old remedy has no effect on nails whatsoever.

❖ Obesity

At any given time, one out of every six Americans is on a weight-loss diet—and for good reason. While much of the world goes hungry, nearly half the American population is overweight or obese. Being obese (weighing 20 percent or more over your desirable weight) has numerous serious health consequences. Cancers of the breast, uterus, and ovaries are more common in obese women; cancers of the colon, rectum, and prostate are more common in obese men. Heart disease, respiratory problems, arthritis, gallbladder disease, and menstrual problems are all more likely if you are obese, and people who are overweight or obese are much more likely to develop adult-onset diabetes.

To determine a patient's ideal weight, physicians often use this basic rule of thumb: For men, they allow 106 pounds for the first five feet of height, then add six pounds for every inch over that. For women, they allow 100 pounds for the first five feet, then add five pounds for every inch over that. This formula doesn't take body type into consideration, however. Because bones and muscles weigh more than fat, someone with a slender frame will weigh less than someone who is the same height but has a huskier frame or more muscles.

No one can tell you what the exact right weight is for you. Some researchers would argue that the weight guideline given above is unrealistically low and doesn't make enough allowance for body type and age. Some recent research suggests, for example, that most people can get a little heavier as they grow older without added risk to their health while other research contradicts this. The chart on the next page gives suggested weight ranges for adults based on studies by the National Research Council of the National Academy of Sciences. If your weight for your height falls within the guidelines of the chart, you probably are at or near a healthy weight for you.

How can you achieve your ideal weight? The answer is easy: Eat less and exercise more. As a first step, you need to determine how many calories a day are right for you. Again, a simple rule of thumb can be used for both men and women: You need 10 calories for every pound of body weight to meet your basic metabolic needs. To this, add 3 calories per pound for your normal daily activities. A woman who weighs 120 pounds, for example, would need to consume, 1,560 calories a day to maintain her weight, but if she became regularly more active while eating the same number of calories, she would lose weight. If she consistently ate less and was also more active, she would lose weight faster.

Suggested Weights for Adults

Height	Weight in Pounds	
	19–34 Years	35 Years and Older
5'0"	97–128	108–138
5'1"	101–132	111–143
5'2"	104–137	115–148
5'3"	107–141	119–152
5'4"	111–146	122–157
5'5"	114–150	126–162
5'6"	118–155	130–167
5'7"	121 160	134–172
5'8"	125–164	138–178
5'9"	129–169	142–183
5'10"	132–174	146–188
5'11"	136–179	151–194
6'0"	140–184	155–199
6'1"	144–189	159–205
6'2"	148–195	164–210
6'3"	152–200	168–216
6'4"	156–205	173–222

Note: Assumes height without shoes and weight without clothes. The higher weights in the ranges generally apply to men, who tend to have more muscle and heavier bones; the lower weights generally apply to women, who tend to have less muscle and lighter bones.

An important first step toward losing weight is paying attention to what you eat in the course of a typical day. Most people seriously underestimate how many calories they take in, and tend to overestimate how many calories exercise burns off. Experts in weight control usually suggest that you begin a weight-loss program by keeping a food diary. Write down everything you eat and drink in the course of a day, and continue the diary for several weeks. Use the diary to discover the hidden calories you are consuming and find ways to cut back without feeling deprived. For example, since putting two tablespoons of creamy blue cheese dressing on your healthful, low-calorie salad adds about 150 calories, you could easily cut back on the amount of dressing. Other calorie-cutting ideas include having iced tea or plain seltzer instead of a sugary soft drink. Substitute fresh fruit for cookies, potato chips, and other high-calorie snack foods.

In general, a good weight-loss diet is the same as a good, healthful diet for anyone: high in fiber, low in fat, with lots of fresh fruits, fresh vegetables, and whole grains. Read more about the basics of a healthful diet in the introduction of this book. To make a quick change from the diet that has made you obese, however, try some of these tips:

- Avoid the empty calories and bad health effects of junk foods and alcoholic beverages.
- Reduce the amount of fat in your diet. Try to get no more than 25 percent of your daily calories from fat.
- Replace fatty or high-protein foods with carbohydrates. Have an extra whole wheat roll or two instead of another piece of fried chicken.
- Enjoy a healthful appetizer with lunch or dinner. Try having a piece of melon or grapefruit, a glass of fruit juice, a small bowl of soup, a salad, or some other appetizer to start a meal. You'll probably eat less of the main course and may not even have room for dessert.
- Eat more often. This may seem paradoxical, but eating several small, low-calorie, low-fat meals throughout the day could be better for you than eating three larger meals. You won't get as hungry between meals and you won't feel deprived.
- Avoid foods that are heavily sweetened, even if they use a noncaloric artificial sweetener. Sweet foods, even noncaloric ones, can make you feel hungrier. That doesn't mean you can never have anything sweet again. Try eating fresh fruit or unsweetened fruit juices instead of cookies or candy. Even a toasted English muffin with a spoonful of jam (no butter) has about 100 fewer calories than a slice of chocolate cake.

- Drink plenty of fluids—six to eight glasses a day.
- Consider joining a weight-loss program such as Weight Watchers. The group support and nutritional education in these programs can be very helpful.

There are no magic powders, pills, or other potions that lead to instant weight loss. Crash diets that promise you will lose ten pounds in just one week, fad diets that restrict you to certain foods, and very low-calorie diets that allow only liquid nutrition may indeed lead to temporary, short-term weight loss. These diets inevitably fail in the long run and may even be dangerous to your health. Yo-yo dieting, where you rapidly lose weight and just as rapidly gain it back, simply makes it even harder to lose weight later. In the end, large fluctuations in weight may be more detrimental to your health than remaining overweight. A more healthful approach is to permanently modify your eating habits and get more exercise. Long-term, permanent weight loss is a slow but steady process. Most doctors agree that losing just a pound a week is a realistic goal.

❖ Osteoporosis

After you reach age thirty-five, your bones gradually begin to lose mass. As the years go by, this could lead to osteoporosis: thin, brittle bones that fracture easily. Osteoporosis is the leading cause of bone fractures in postmenopausal women and the elderly. Over 1.3 million osteoporosis-related fractures occur each year in the United States, primarily of the hip, spine, and wrist. The cost to society is estimated at $7 to $10 billion.

Osteoporosis can't be cured, but it can be prevented or slowed down by including enough calcium in your diet. Although calcium is essential for building and maintaining strong bones (your body contains about three pounds of it), according to the National Institutes of Health, only half the children and young adults in America are getting their optimal calcium intake: between 1,200 and 1,500 milligrams a day. By some other estimates, eight out of ten American women don't get enough calcium. The NIH now recommends that women age twenty-five to fifty and men age twenty-five to sixty-five get 1,000 milligrams of calcium daily. (In addition to helping prevent osteoporosis, there is some evidence that this level of calcium may also protect you against developing high blood pressure.)

Some people have a genetic predisposition to osteoporosis. It is much more common among women than men. White women are more likely to develop osteoporosis than black women. Thin, petite women are more susceptible, as are those with a family history of osteoporosis.

Menopausal women are at particular risk for osteoporosis. This is because their decreased estrogen levels cause bone loss to be accelerated for a period of about six to eight years; after that, bone loss becomes more gradual. To lower the risk, doctors now recommend that menopausal women get 1,000 to 1,500 milligrams of calcium daily. Both men and women over the age of sixty-five should aim for 1,500 milligrams daily.

The best way to get enough calcium is through diet. Milk is the best dietary source of calcium: one 8-ounce glass of nonfat milk has about 300 milligrams of calcium. Other good sources of dietary calcium include such dairy products as yogurt and cheese, almonds, broccoli, dark green leafy vegetables, tofu (bean curd), sardines and canned salmon (with the bones), oatmeal, and kidney beans. Even so, it's hard to get enough calcium through diet alone, especially if you can't tolerate milk. If you feel you're not getting enough calcium, try some of the new calcium-fortified fruit juices, cereals, and breads now available. Most daily multivitamin supplements include calcium. If you are pregnant or nursing, or if you are menopausal, discuss calcium supplements with your doctor. Most physicians recommend supplements that contain calcium carbonate. Menopausal women should also discuss estrogen replacement therapy, since this has been shown to significantly reduce the risk of fractures.

To use calcium properly, you also need adequate levels of vitamin D. Your body produces its own vitamin D from exposure to sunlight and also gets it from your diet. As you age, your body's ability to make its own vitamin D is reduced, so it's especially important for you to get the recommended 400 IU a day. Good dietary sources of vitamin D are cod liver oil, fortified milk, egg yolks, tuna, salmon, canned sardines, shrimp, and liver. Bear in mind that most dairy products are not made with fortified milk and are not good sources of vitamin D. You can also take supplemental vitamin D, but this can be toxic at high levels. Discuss supplements with your doctor before you use them.

Certain drugs, such as aluminum antacids, cortisone, thyroxine, and some antibiotics, may accelerate bone loss. If you need to take drugs of this sort for an extended time, discuss calcium supplements with your doctor

Tobacco, alcohol, and caffeine can interfere with your body's absorption of calcium. If you smoke, stop. Even if you increase your calcium intake, your chances of osteoporosis remain high if you continue to smoke. Cut back on alcohol and caffeine. Osteoporosis in young and middle-aged men is often a result of alcoholism.

Inactivity is a risk factor for osteoporosis, so keep moving as you get older. Weight-bearing exercise, such as walking, jogging, and bike riding, is very helpful for building bone strength and preventing osteoporosis. A brisk daily walk of only twenty or thirty minutes can make a big difference.

See also Menopause.

❖ Parkinson's Disease

A slowly progressive disease generally associated with tremor or trembling of the arms and legs, stiffness and rigidity of the muscles, and slowness of movement, Parkinson's disease affects about one million Americans. Each year, some 50,000 new cases are diagnosed. Parkinson's disease generally affects men and women over the age of forty. Although there is no cure for Parkinson's disease, many patients respond well to drugs and physical therapy.

The cause of Parkinson's disease is unknown, although researchers believe that it is related to a chemical imbalance in the brain. The brains of Parkinson's patients no longer produce a neurotransmitter substance called dopamine. Levodopa, more commonly known as L-dopa, is the primary drug used for treating Parkinson's disease. In combination with another drug, carbidopa (Sinemet is the brand name), L-dopa helps replace some of the missing dopamine and relieve Parkinson's symptoms.

Research over the years has shown that the diet of Parkinson's patients has a lot to do with how well they respond to L-dopa. Today, most doctors recommend that Parkinson's patients eat a protein-restricted diet; when they do eat protein, such as meat, they should eat it only at the evening meal, when they are likely to be less active. This is because digesting protein releases amino acids into the bloodstream. The amino acids then compete with the L-dopa to cross into the brain. The more amino acids in the blood, the less L-dopa gets into the brain, and the less effective the medication will be. Some recent research suggests that this approach could be modified somewhat by keeping the carbohydrate-to-protein ratio of all meals at about seven to one. At that level, the amino acids don't seem to interfere with the L-dopa. In any case, try to be consistent about meals. Eat at about the same time every day and eat about the same amount. Every patient is different in his or her response to L-dopa, and your response can change over time. Discuss any dietary changes carefully with your doctor before making them.

Before Sinemet became part of the standard therapy for Parkinson's, patients were advised to avoid vitamin B_6 in supplements and in such foods as meat, fish, liver, bananas, peanuts, potatoes, wheat germ, beans, avocados, and whole grains. This is no longer necessary. There is no evidence that Parkinson's disease has anything to do with nutritional deficiencies, and there is no evidence that any particular vitamins or minerals help the condition. You may want to take a daily multivitamin supplement, but megadoses of vitamins do not help Parkinson's disease and could be dangerous. High doses of vitamin A and vitamin E, for example, can be toxic.

Chewing and swallowing can be a problem for Parkinson's patients. In such cases, soft foods, purees, milk shakes, puddings, and the like can help ensure good nutrition. Your doctor can refer you to a dietitian for guidance. Another common problem for Parkinson's patients is constipation. As for anyone else, this problem can be reduced or avoided by drinking lots of fluids (six to eight glasses daily) and eating plenty of fresh fruits and vegetables. (See the section on Constipation for more information.)

❖ Pregnancy

At no time in a woman's life is nutrition more important than when she is pregnant, and at no time are the benefits of good nutrition more obvious.

If you're planning a pregnancy, you need to make sure your diet is a good one starting immediately. Being the right weight for your height will increase your chances of conception and make your pregnancy easier. More importantly, your unborn baby is most susceptible to harm two to eight weeks after conception, but you might not know you're pregnant until three or more weeks after conception. If you've been eating right all along, though, the chances of having a healthy baby will be very good.

The United States Public Health Service now advises all women capable of becoming pregnant to consume 0.4 milligrams (400 micrograms) of folic acid daily, either from dietary sources or supplements. Folic acid, also called folacin or folate, is one of the B vitamins. Conclusive evidence now shows that folacin helps prevent neural tube defects in unborn children. Because these defects, which can cause spina bifida, anencephaly, and other crippling problems, develop in the first two weeks after conception, it's vital for women to get enough folic acid *before* they become pregnant.

Folic acid is found in brewer's yeast, asparagus, dark green leafy vegetables, lentils and other cooked dried beans and peas, liver, citrus fruits and juices, peanuts, wheat germ, avocados, beets, broccoli, oatmeal, sunflower seeds, bananas, and whole grains. Many breakfast cereals are also now fortified with folic acid. Although folic acid is found in many foods, if you are planning to get pregnant, you should consider taking supplements. Discuss the question with your doctor, however, before adding supplements to your diet. Folic acid needs vitamin B_{12}, niacin, and vitamin C to be used properly by your body, so you might also want to consider taking a daily multivitamin supplement, especially if you are a vegetarian. Don't take megadoses of vitamins or minerals—these can lead to birth defects.

Women who drink alcohol during pregnancy—even as little as one drink a day—can damage their unborn baby. Fetal alcohol syndrome can lead to mental retardation, poor growth, physical defects, and other problems for your child. If you're planning to become pregnant or already are, avoid alcohol. You should also avoid taking drugs of any sort, if possible. Recreational drugs such as cocaine and marijuana can cause miscarriage, premature birth, and birth defects.

Recent studies have found that caffeine in moderation is safe for pregnant women. You can consume up to 300 milligrams a day—that's the equivalent of three 8-ounce cups of coffee, seven 8-ounce cups of tea, or five 12-ounce cans of cola.

If you take any prescription drugs and are planning a pregnancy, discuss the situation with your doctor. Some nonprescription drugs could have an adverse effect on your baby. Try to avoid these products altogether if you are planning to get pregnant. If you already are, speak to your doctor before taking any over-the-counter medicine. Even aspirin can cause problems, especially in the first three months of pregnancy.

Once you've become pregnant, you'll need to take in enough extra calories to nourish you both—and the best way to do that is through a good, nutritious diet. Eating right will help your baby grow and will also help you feel your best. Pregnant women should follow the basic guidelines of the food pyramid (see the first part of this book for more information). Limit fatty foods, sweets, and junk-food snacks. Skip junk food in favor of quality snacks such as fresh fruit, crackers with peanut butter, or yogurt.

In general, during the first three months of pregnancy, you need to eat about 150 additional calories a day; after that, you should aim for 350 extra calories a day. Most doctors recommend that you gain about twenty-five to thirty-five pounds during your pregnancy (if you're having twins, you should gain about forty pounds). Today, doctors worry more about women who gain too little weight than those who gain too much, since inadequate nutrition during pregnancy can lead to a baby with mental retardation or other problems. Don't diet while you're pregnant!

Along with the extra calories, pregnant women need to increase their intake of protein, folic acid, vitamin B_6, vitamin B_{12}, and vitamin C. They also need about 400 extra milligrams of calcium a day and 30 to 60 milligrams a day of extra iron. Good sources of protein in the diet are meat, poultry, fish, and cheese. Simply add an ounce or two more to your serving at each meal. Good sources of folic acid are discussed above; the B vitamins are found in whole grains, liver, bananas, chicken, avocados, peanuts, and cooked dried beans and peas. Vitamin C is found in citrus fruits and juices, strawberries and other fresh fruits, dark green leafy vegetables, and cruciferous vegetables, including cauliflower, broccoli, and brussels sprouts. You can get extra calcium by drinking more milk or eating more yogurt, cheese, and other dairy products; other good dietary sources of calcium are broccoli, tofu, canned salmon, and dark green leafy vegetables, such as kale and chard. Iron is found in red meat, organ meats, seafood and shellfish, nuts, spinach, and whole grains. To be on the safe side, your doctor will probably recommend that you eat plenty of fresh fruits and vegetables and also prescribe vitamin and mineral supplements, especially iron and calcium supplements.

Eating properly can help relieve some of the common discomforts of being pregnant. For example, many women become constipated during pregnancy. Getting lots of dietary fiber and drinking plenty of fluids can help relieve this problem as well as help prevent hemorrhoids. Heartburn is another common problem for pregnant women. Try eating several small meals a day instead of three larger ones; avoid spicy or greasy foods and foods you know don't agree with you; skip carbonated beverages and coffee; and don't lie down immediately after eating. Again, refrain from taking over-the-counter antacids or anything else without your doctor's approval.

Some fluid retention, or edema, is common and normal in pregnancy. But since edema can be a symptom of a serious condition called toxemia, tell your doctor at once if you notice that your hands, legs, feet, or face are getting swollen or puffy. You can help relieve the discomfort of mild fluid retention by cutting back on salt and resting with your legs elevated.

No woman gets through a pregnancy without hearing innumerable jokes about food cravings. Some women do indeed get sudden cravings for foods such as ice cream, but much more common is a desire for salty foods. This probably happens because pregnant women do need more sodium. Some women may develop cravings for unusual substances such as clay or cornstarch. This condition, called pica, is probably caused by an iron deficiency. If you have pica, tell your doctor. And as a general rule, if it's not food, don't eat it.

See also Breast-Feeding; Infertility; Morning Sickness.

❖ Premenstrual Syndrome (PMS)

Premenstrual syndrome, better known as PMS, refers to a variety of symptoms that women can experience one to two weeks before the start of their menstrual periods. Over 150 PMS symptoms have been identified, but most fall into four groups:

- Nervous tension, irritability, anxiety, mood swings
- Weight gain, swelling of hands or feet, breast tenderness, abdominal bloating
- Headache, craving for sweets, increased appetite, pounding heart, fatigue, dizziness, fainting
- Depression, forgetfulness, crying, confusion, insomnia

PMS symptoms occur before a woman's period begins; they generally improve once the period has started. PMS symptoms should not be confused with menstrual cramps and other problems—PMS has a different cause and treatment.

Somewhat less than half of all women have PMS to some degree. For most, the symptoms are minor inconveniences and can be dealt with easily. For about 10 percent of PMS sufferers, however, the symptoms can be a real problem, interfering with family relationships and work.

The exact causes of PMS are still unknown, but some research suggests that diet plays a role. Some women find that increasing their intake of vitamin B_6 and magnesium can help relieve their symptoms, although why this sometimes helps is still not understood. Foods that are high in vitamin B_6 include brewer's yeast, bananas, avocados, green peppers, walnuts, cantaloupe, cabbage, dark green leafy vegetables, pecans, peanuts, soybeans, wheat germ, and egg yolks. Magnesium is found in milk, buckwheat, millet, cashews, almonds, peanuts, spinach, carrots, and wheat bran. Discuss supplements of vitamin B_6, magnesium, and other vitamins and minerals with your doctor before trying them.

In general, eating a well-balanced diet that is low in fat, high in fiber, and has lots of fresh fruits and vegetables will improve your overall nutritional status and may also help relieve some PMS symptoms. Many women find that eating six small meals a day on a regular schedule, rather than three larger ones, helps keep their energy levels steady. Eating complex carbohydrates such as beans, pasta, whole grains, and the like can also help; in general, avoid sugar and fat. If you tend to retain fluid as part of your PMS, try limiting your salt intake in the days before your period. Cutting back on caffeine could relieve tension, insomnia, and breast tenderness. Avoid alcohol, since it has depressant effects.

See also Menstrual Cramps.

❖ Prostate Disease

An important gland in the male reproductive system, the prostate is located in front of the rectum and just below the bladder. Roughly the size and shape of a walnut, the prostate gland is wrapped around the urethra, the tube that carries urine from the bladder out through the penis. After a man reaches age forty, and especially after the age of sixty, the prostate may become a source of problems.

Prostate cancer is the most common major cancer in American men, occurring in one out of ten. In its early stages, it has no symptoms. When detected at that point, it can usually be cured.

Recent research has pointed to a link between a high-fat diet and advanced prostate cancer. For example, black men living in west Africa eat a low-fat diet and have very low rates of prostate cancer. African-American men, on the other hand, have a high rate of prostate cancer and tend to eat a lot of saturated fats. Animal fat may be the real culprit. Current dietary recommendations suggest that everyone get less than 30 percent of their daily calories from fat. If you are worried about prostate cancer, think about cutting back on fat to the recommended level or below.

A link may exist between phytoestrogens, hormonelike compounds found in some foods, and prostate cancer. Isoflavonoids, a type of phytoestrogen found in beans, peas, lentils, and dried fruits, may help protect against prostate cancer. Japanese men, who eat lots of tofu (made from soybeans) have a low rate of prostate cancer. The vitamin A and beta carotene found in dark green leafy vegetables and orange or yellow vegetables, such as carrots and squash, may also have a protective effect.

Benign prostatic hyperplasia (BPH), or enlarged prostate, is a condition that eventually develops in about 80 percent of all men. When the prostate gland enlarges, it squeezes the urethra, which can sometimes cause difficulty in urinating or other urinary tract problems. Enlarged prostate is not cancer and does not lead to cancer.

Some men have found that adding zinc to their diet can help relieve BPH symptoms. Good dietary sources of zinc include oysters, dark-meat turkey, liver, lima beans, pumpkin seeds, and wheat germ. Discuss zinc supplements with your doctor before trying them, however. If you have BPH, it is important to drink plenty of fluids and empty your bladder fully when you urinate. This will help prevent bladder infections.

❖ Psoriasis

A persistent skin disease that causes inflammation, scaling, and itchiness, psoriasis affects millions of people. The cause is unknown, but it may be that an abnormality in the functioning of certain white cells in the blood triggers the skin inflammation. This causes the skin to shed itself too rapidly—in three or four days, instead of the usual thirty.

Psoriasis usually begins with little red bumps on the skin. These gradually grow larger and scales form. The top scales flake off easily, but the scales below cause red, itchy patches on the skin. The elbows, knees, groin and genitals, arms, legs, scalp, and nails are the areas most commonly affected.

People with severe psoriasis often get desperate enough to try quack remedies and strange diets. There is no evidence that removing yeast or dairy products from your diet or taking megadoses of lecithin or other vitamins and minerals will help your psoriasis. One type of synthetic vitamin D does help some psoriasis patients, but it must be prescribed by your doctor. Eating foods high in vitamin D is not a substitute for this medication. Sunshine, which helps your body synthesize its own vitamin D, does help psoriasis. Your doctor can advise you about the use of a sunlamp.

Fish oil aids the body in the manufacture of eicosapentanoic acid (EPA), which in large amounts has helped reduce itching and inflammation for some psoriasis patients. To get enough EPA to see results, you will probably have to take supplements. Discuss this with your doctor before trying it.

For temporary relief of itching, try a soothing colloidal oatmeal bath. You can purchase colloidal oatmeal (Aveeno brand) at the drugstore, or make it yourself by grinding ordinary rolled oats in a food processor until they are a fine powder. Put two cups into a tub of lukewarm water and soak for twenty minutes or so.

❖ Radiation Therapy

Half of all cancer patients receive radiation therapy. In fact, for many patients, radiation is the only treatment needed. Radiation is sometimes used to shrink tumors before they are removed surgically. In other cases, radiation is used to relieve cancer symptoms. Unfortunately, radiation therapy can have unpleasant side effects, although these can usually be managed with medication and careful attention to diet.

Good nutrition is a must because it helps damaged tissues rebuild themselves. Patients who eat well tolerate the therapy better and recover more quickly. But side effects of radiation, such as loss of appetite, nausea, and discomfort from chewing and swallowing, can keep patients from eating enough. Modern antiemetic drugs can be a big help for those suffering from nausea. Discuss these drugs with your doctor before beginning therapy, and follow the tips below for good eating.

To cope with loss of appetite, eat when you are hungry. Try having several small meals a day instead of three larger ones. Keep nutritious snacks on hand to nibble on if you feel hungry but don't want much. Choose foods that taste good to you and that are easy to eat. If you can eat only a small amount at one time, make sure you get the maximum number of calories you can from the meal. Try adding cream or milk to canned cream soups instead of water. Eggnog, milk shakes, or prepared liquid supplements are tasty, nutritious, and easy to swallow. Cream sauce, butter, or melted cheese on your vegetables will add calories and flavor. If you can't handle solid foods, drink plenty of nutritious liquids. Try adding powdered nonfat milk, plain yogurt, honey, or prepared liquid supplements to your drinks.

If you are having radiation to the head or neck area, you may have redness and irritation in the mouth, dry mouth, difficulty in swallowing, changes in taste, or nausea. You still need to eat, however. Avoid spices and coarse foods, such as raw vegetables, dry crackers, and nuts. Don't drink alcohol, and avoid sugary foods. If your mouth is dry, sip cool water throughout the day; some patients find that carbonated beverages help relieve dry mouth better than plain water. Sugar-free candy or gum may also help. Moisten foods with sauces or gravy to make eating them easier. It's very important to take proper care of your teeth during this time. Your doctor will work with you and your dentist to help you with dental care.

Radiation therapy in the chest area can make swallowing difficult or painful. Try mashing or pureeing your foods or adding gravies or sauces to make them softer. Avoid foods that are dry and rough, such as crackers or nuts. Cut foods into small, bite-sized pieces. Discuss liquid food supplements with your doctor if solid food is too uncomfortable to eat.

Nausea, vomiting, and diarrhea can be serious problems for patients who are getting radiation to the stomach and abdomen. If you feel nauseous after a treatment, try not eating for several hours before the next treatment. Some patients handle the radiation better on an empty stomach. After your treatment, you may find it helpful to wait one or two hours before eating again. If your doctor or dietitian prescribes a special diet, try to stick to it. To deal with nausea, eat six or more small meals or snacks throughout the day rather than three larger ones. Avoid foods that are fried, fatty, or have a strong smell. Drink plenty of cool liquids between meals. After three or four weeks of radiation therapy, you may develop diarrhea. To deal with this, your doctor may prescribe medication and some changes in your diet. Try a clear liquid diet as soon as the diarrhea starts or you feel it might start. Water, apple juice, peach nectar, plain gelatin, clear broth, and weak tea are all good. Avoid milk and milk products and foods that are high in fiber. When the diarrhea starts to improve, try eating small amounts of low-fiber foods such as bananas, cottage cheese, rice, applesauce, mashed potatoes, and dry toast. Have foods that are high in potassium, such as bananas, potatoes, avocados, orange juice, and apricots, since you may lose a lot of this mineral from diarrhea.

Fortunately, the side effects of radiation therapy go away once the therapy stops. For most people, radiation therapy is given five days a week for six or seven weeks. It may take some time after that, however, for your appetite and strength to return fully.

See also Chemotherapy.

❖ Raynaud's Disease

Raynaud's disease causes the small arteries that supply blood to your fingers to become supersensitive to cold. When exposed to cold air, these small blood vessels suddenly contract, reducing the flow of blood to your hands and leaving your fingers pale or bluish and numb. The condition is temporary, however, and normal color and feeling return once you warm up your hands. (Feet may sometimes be affected, too.) Raynaud's disease is quite common. It usually affects women, starting in early adulthood. Occasionally, it can be traced to an underlying problem, such as scleroderma or working with heavy power tools such as pneumatic drills, but generally there is no known cause. Over the course of many years, Raynaud's disease can at worst lead to weakened fingers and a diminished sense of touch, but generally it is more of an annoyance than a serious problem.

Self-help can do a lot to relieve the symptoms of Raynaud's disease. If you smoke, stop. Smoking further constricts the small blood vessels and makes your circulation worse. Dress warmly in cold weather. Wear loose, comfortable layers of clothing, warm socks, warm gloves or mittens, and a hat. Hot foods and drinks can help keep you warm in cold weather, but avoid coffee, tea, and other beverages with caffeine, since the caffeine can constrict your blood vessels. Avoid alcoholic beverages. The alcohol temporarily opens the blood vessels in your hands and feet and may make them feel warmer for a few minutes, but ultimately this causes your core body temperature to drop and blood flow to your extremities will be further reduced.

Because omega-3 fatty acids (fish oil) can improve circulation, you might try adding more deep-sea fish such as tuna, mackerel, and herring to your diet, or try a daily fish oil capsule; however, don't take fish oil capsules if you're diabetic.

❖ Restless Leg Syndrome

Just as some people are trying to fall asleep, they start to feel a crawling or twitching sensation in their legs, especially the thighs, and they have a strong urge to move their legs. This annoying but not dangerous condition, called restless leg syndrome, is most common in middle-aged and older people; about 5 percent of the population suffers from it. Occasionally, the symptoms are an indication of a more serious problem such as diabetes, Parkinson's disease, or kidney disease, however, so see your doctor if you suddenly develop the problem or if it gets much worse. Pregnant women also sometimes get restless leg syndrome, but it usually goes away after the baby is born.

Sometimes restless leg syndrome clears up if you take supplemental iron, calcium, folic acid, or vitamin E. Try taking a daily multivitamin. Eating a large meal shortly before bedtime worsens symptoms for some patients. Others find that caffeine makes their legs more restless. Exercise such as walking before bedtime seems to help. Some people swear that taking a hot bath before bed helps, while others claim that cold soaks work for them. Every case of restless leg syndrome seems to be different, so experiment until you find techniques that best help you.

❖ Rosacea

When you blush, the skin on your face, especially your cheeks, turns red. If you have rosacea, a disease affecting the skin of the face, the same areas that turn red when you blush are red all the time. Later, pimples and red lines from enlarged blood vessels appear. If rosacea isn't treated, some people—especially men—may get small, knobby bumps on the nose. As more bumps appear, your nose looks swollen and red. Rosacea, not alcoholism, is why the comedian W.C. Fields had a large, red nose.

Despite the pimples, which resemble teenage acne, rosacea is a disease of adults. It seems to affect fair-skinned people more often, although people with any skin type can get it. People who blush or flush easily are more likely to get rosacea.

In most people, rosacea is a chronic condition that comes and goes in cycles. It often responds well to medications that treat the pimples. Facial flushing can make rosacea symptoms flare up. Stress, sunlight, exercise, and extreme heat or cold can lead to flushing. So can hot drinks, caffeine, alcohol, and spicy foods. All are to be avoided if possible. Sometimes a particular food can cause a flare-up. Culprits can include fruits, dairy products, and chocolate. If you have an episode of rosacea that you can't trace to heat or some other cause, suspect a food.

❖ Shingles

Anyone who's had chicken pox (and most people have it as children) could develop shingles, an unpleasant ailment characterized by pain and skin blisters. The reason is that both diseases are caused by the same herpes zoster virus, which can remain dormant in certain nerve cells in your body and then reactivate later in life. About 20 percent of the population will get shingles at some point, although it is more likely to occur in people over age fifty.

An attack of shingles generally begins with burning pain or tingling and extreme sensitivity in one area of the skin.

After a few days, a red rash erupts and soon turns into blisters that resemble chicken pox. The blisters usually last for two to three weeks, then crust over and begin to disappear. The severe pain that goes with them may last longer. The blisters of shingles are most common on the trunk and buttocks. Sometimes blisters appear on the face or nose, which is cause for serious concern, because if the blisters should involve the eye region, permanent eye damage can result. If you have shingles and develop blisters on the face, see an eye doctor at once. Sometimes older people who have had shingles develop postherpetic neuralgia, a complication where the pain of shingles continues long after the blisters have gone away.

Shingles is far less contagious than chicken pox, but someone who has shingles may transmit chicken pox to someone who has never had it. If you have shingles, avoid contact with very young children, pregnant women, and people whose immune systems are depressed, such as cancer or AIDS patients.

Most people who have shingles get better in a few weeks without medication, although your doctor may prescribe the antiviral drug acyclovir to help speed the process. To treat the symptoms, doctors recommend calamine lotion, cold compresses, soothing baths in colloidal oatmeal, and painkillers such as ibuprofen. You can purchase colloidal oatmeal (Aveeno brand) at the drugstore, or make it yourself by grinding ordinary rolled oats in a food processor until they are a fine powder. Put two cups into a tub of lukewarm water and soak for twenty minutes or so.

The herpes zoster virus is related to the herpes virus that causes cold sores and genital herpes. It is possible that eating foods containing the amino acid arginine could worsen your shingles symptoms. Foods that are high in arginine include chocolate, nuts of all sorts, peanuts, seeds, grains, gelatin, brussels sprouts, and coconut. The amino acid lysine seems to inhibit the herpes virus. Some shingles sufferers find that supplemental lysine, available in capsules at health food stores, helps relieve their symptoms. Try 500 milligrams a day until the symptoms go away.

See also Cold Sores; Herpes.

❖ Sinusitis

Sinuses are cavities in the cheekbones found around and behind your nose. The cavities are lined with mucus membranes, just as the insides of your nostrils are. Your sinuses play an important role in warming and moisturizing the air that enters the nasal cavity. If the membranes lining your sinuses become inflamed, they swell up and close off the narrow passages that connect the sinuses to the nasal cavity. When you get sinusitis, infected material builds up inside the sinus cavities, causing the most common sinusitis symptom, a severe headache. Other symptoms of sinusitis include coughing, tiredness, stuffy nose, bad breath, bad-tasting postnasal drip, and thick, colored mucus.

Sinusitis often develops after you have had a cold and goes away by itself after a week or so. Some people have chronic sinusitis as a result of allergies or a structural abnormality of the sinuses. Depending on the cause, your doctor may prescribe antibiotics, decongestants, or painkillers to relieve the symptoms. If your sinusitis is caused by allergies, your doctor will probably refer you to an allergist to explore how the allergies can be treated.

You can also take some useful self-help steps to relieve the discomfort of sinusitis. Drink plenty of liquids—six to eight glasses of water, juice, broth, and the like—every day. This helps thin the mucus and makes it easier to expel. Chicken soup can be helpful because it contains the amino acid cysteine, which thins mucus. Spicy foods containing garlic, cayenne pepper, or horseradish act as natural decongestants. Sleeping with a cold mist vaporizer is often helpful. If you smoke, stop. Cigarette smoke is very irritating to the sinuses. Avoid alcohol as well. It can make the symptoms worse and could also interact badly with any prescription medicines you are taking.

See also Allergies.

❖ Skin Cancer

Having a glowing tan may give the illusion of health, but in the long run, the ultraviolet rays in sunlight can lead to premature wrinkles and skin cancer. Today, skin cancer is very common. Over the course of your lifetime, your risk of getting melanoma is now one in a hundred and may be rising.

Three types of skin cancer are of particular concern: basal cell carcinoma, squamous cell carcinoma, and melanoma. Those at greatest risk for these cancers are fair-skinned, have red or blond hair, sunburn easily, or work or play outside a lot. Having a lot of freckles or moles is another risk factor.

Skin cancer is easy to detect and can usually be completely cured if caught early. Check yourself for skin cancer with the ABCDE rule:

- **A**symmetry: moles that aren't circular
- **B**order: moles that have jagged or blurry edges
- **C**olor: moles that darken, change color, or lose color
- **D**iameter: moles that are larger than a quarter of an inch across
- **E**levation: moles that are raised above the skin and have an uneven surface

If you notice any of the above signs, you could have skin cancer, especially if you are over age thirty. Other signs include moles that bleed, grow rapidly, or itch. Any persistent area of irritated skin or sore that doesn't heal could also be cancerous. See your doctor at once.

Prevention is the best approach to skin cancer. Your best defense is to avoid excessive sunlight exposure by staying out of the sun or using a sunblocking lotion with an SPF (sun protection factor) of 15 or greater. Avoid tanning booths and sunlamps. Although these may claim to be safe because they use only "harmless" UVA rays that don't cause cancer, this is not true.

Besides avoiding the sun, it is possible that diet can play a role in preventing skin cancer. Some evidence suggests that omega-6 fatty acids, found in safflower oil, corn oil, and sunflower oil, may encourage the growth of skin cancer, while omega-3 fatty acids, found in deep-sea fish such as tuna and halibut, may inhibit it.

❖ Skin Care
See Acne; Dry Skin; Sunburn.

❖ Smoking

Cigarette smoking, a cause of lung cancer, heart disease, emphysema, and chronic bronchitis, among other fatal illnesses, is directly responsible for the deaths of 400,000

Americans every year, and indirectly responsible for still more deaths and illness. Since cigarette smoking is guaranteed to cause health problems, the question is, why is anyone still smoking?

The answer is that the nicotine in tobacco smoke is an addictive drug, and addictions are hard to break. If you are truly motivated to quit, however, you can. Here are some hints from the American Lung Association:

- Set a target date for quitting.
- Keep a smoking diary. If you know when and why you smoke, you can change your habits more easily.
- Smoke fewer cigarettes each day as you approach your target date.
- Postpone the urge for a cigarette. If you wait even five minutes after the urge strikes, it will probably pass without your lighting up.
- Chew sugarless gum instead of smoking.
- Buy only one pack of cigarettes at a time.

Many people worry that they will gain weight when they stop smoking, and they probably will. But usually the amount gained is only five to ten pounds. The health risks of being five or even fifteen pounds heavier are trivial compared to the health risks of smoking. If you gain a lot of weight after quitting cigarettes, take the next step toward healthy living and examine your diet. Use the confidence you gained from beating a difficult habit to make some changes.

One school of thought claims that a high-acid diet flushes nicotine from the system faster. The drawback is that the urge to smoke increases as your body is depleted of the nicotine it craves. On the other hand, if you can steel yourself to the cravings and want to get rid of the nicotine in your body, acidity could help you get over the withdrawal symptoms more quickly. Some ex-smokers swear that drinking a lot of citrus juice, which is high in acid, for a couple of weeks after they quit helped them get through that difficult time. Taking 1,000 milligrams a day of vitamin C seems to have a similar effect.

❖ Sore Throat

A scratchy feeling in your throat is annoying but most often isn't serious. Sore throats might have many causes: a cold or flu, hay fever, smoking too much, or breathing smoky or polluted air. On the other hand, if you have a sore throat along with high fever, headache, pain when you swallow, and sore glands in your jaw and throat, you might have tonsillitis, strep throat, or mononucleosis. If you think your sore throat is caused by one of these illnesses, see your doctor soon.

Some old-fashioned remedies for relieving a sore throat are still favorites today. You could try gargling with warm water and salt or lemon juice (1 teaspoon to 8 ounces of water). Repeat several times a day. In general, drinking a lot of fluids will help ease your sore throat by keeping the tissues moist. Herbal teas, water, and fruit juices are all good choices, but avoid acidic juices such as orange juice. Many people find that lukewarm beverages are best, but cold or hot ones may feel better to you. Honey, lemon, and tea make a soothing combination. For a more potent mixture, try substituting fresh grated horseradish for the lemon. Sucking on a hard candy or a lozenge can be helpful. Frozen desserts like ice pops or sherbet go down easily and can have a temporary numbing effect. Avoid hard, scratchy foods such as chips, nuts, and crackers. Instead, try soft foods such as bananas, applesauce, puddings, soup, and gelatin.

See also Colds.

❖ Stomach Cancer

The incidence of stomach cancer in the United States has dropped sharply over the past fifty years. The reason is probably an important change in eating habits. Because of modern refrigeration and freezing, we now eat far fewer smoked, salted, or pickled foods—foods that have been directly linked to stomach cancer.

Stomach cancer is difficult to detect early and hard to treat later on. Many of the symptoms, such as indigestion, heartburn, nausea, diarrhea, and loss of appetite, resemble those of stomach viruses or ulcers, among many other problems.

The most common treatment for stomach cancer is surgery to remove some or all of the stomach. After undergoing this sort of surgery, you will need to follow a special diet for at least several weeks and possibly longer. If your stomach has been completely removed, you can no longer absorb vitamin B_{12} and will need to have regular injections of this essential nutrient instead. Your doctor and dietitian will work with you to help you adjust your diet.

To help prevent stomach cancer, eat smoked, salted, and pickled foods in moderation. Avoid nitrites and nitrates, which are often added to foods such as salami, hot dogs, and lunch meats as preservatives. In general, eat a low-fat, high-fiber diet rich in whole grains and fresh fruits and vegetables. It's particularly important to eat vegetables that are high in beta carotene. Orange and yellow vegetables such as carrots, squash, and sweet potatoes are high in beta carotene, as are cantaloupes and apricots. Among the green vegetables, spinach and broccoli are good choices.

See also Chemotherapy; Radiation Therapy.

❖ Stroke and Stroke Prevention

Although stroke is still the third-largest cause of death in America today, stroke deaths have been dropping in recent years. The reason is improved medical care for stroke victims and better treatment for high blood pressure. Even so, the stroke death rate could be lowered far more if more people were to follow stroke prevention dietary guidelines.

A stroke occurs when one of the blood vessels to the brain bursts or become clogged. The rupture or blockage keeps the brain from getting the blood flow it needs. As a result, it starts to die. The stroke can result in severe losses in mental and bodily functions or even death.

The warning signals of stroke are easy to detect. If you notice any of the symptoms below, get medical attention at once:

- Sudden weakness, numbness, or paralysis of the face, arm, and leg, especially on one side of the body.
- Sudden dimness or loss of vision, particularly in one eye.
- Loss of speech or trouble talking or understanding speech.
- Dizziness, unsteadiness, or sudden falls, especially along with any of the above symptoms.

A stroke is a medical emergency. Call 911 for help at once if you suspect a stroke. Stroke-related brain damage gets worse the longer the stroke goes untreated.

About 10 percent of all strokes are preceded by a warning sign called a transient ischemic attack (TIA) that occurs days or even weeks before a major stroke. TIAs occur when a blood clot temporarily blocks an artery and cuts off the blood supply to the brain for a short time. TIAs usually last from only a few minutes to a few hours. The symptoms are the same as for stroke, but they generally go away within twenty-four hours. If you experience a TIA, you are likely to have a stroke soon. See your doctor at once.

Some of the risk factors for stroke are beyond your control, such as simply getting older, being a man, and being an African-American. People with diabetes are also more likely to have strokes, so it's important to keep your diabetes under control. If you've already had a stroke, you are likely to have another one, and you are a good candidate for a stroke if you have high blood pressure and don't control the problem.

Some risk factors can be controlled by changing your lifestyle and diet. If your blood cholesterol is too high, if you smoke, if you drink large amounts of alcohol, and if you are obese, your chances of a stroke are high. (Ways to control each of these risk factors are discussed elsewhere in this book.)

Recent research indicates that you can use diet to help reduce your chances of having a stroke. Even if you don't have high blood pressure, it's probably a good idea to cut back on your salt intake. Beta carotene and vitamin A may have a strong preventive effect by helping to keep cholesterol from building up in your arteries and leading to a blockage. If you do have a stroke, the antioxidant powers of these nutrients may keep the damage from being as severe. Another nutrient that may help ward off strokes is potassium. This could be because potassium helps keep your blood vessels elastic and your blood pressure at normal levels. Conveniently, many of the foods that are rich in beta carotenes are also rich in potassium. These include orange vegetables such as carrots, sweet potatoes, squash, and pumpkin, dark green leafy vegetables such as spinach, kale, and beet greens, and fruits such as apricots, oranges, and cantaloupes.

Including omega-3 fatty acids (fish oil) in your diet might be another good way to reduce your stroke risk. Fish oil could help thin your blood, reducing your chances of a blood clot blocking the flow to your brain. The best dietary source of omega-3 fatty acids is deep-sea fish such as tuna, mackerel, and herring. Try to eat fish instead of beef or other red meat three times a week or more.

If you smoke, stop. If you have more than two alcoholic drinks a day, cut back. Heavy drinking definitely increases your risk of stroke.

See also Diabetes; High Blood Pressure; High Cholesterol; Obesity.

❖ Sunburn

Exposure to the sun's ultraviolet rays can lead to sunburn—skin that is reddened, swollen, or even blistered. At best, sunburn is a painful nuisance; however, a serious sunburn can be extremely uncomfortable and even dangerous.

Cold compresses are helpful for relieving the discomfort of sunburn. Dip a soft cloth in plain cold water and place it on the affected area. Replace the cloth with a fresh one every few minutes, and continue the treatment for ten to fifteen minutes at a time, several times a day. Instead of plain cold water, you could try using a mixture of 1 part milk to 4 parts cold water. Some people claim that compresses of strong, cold tea are effective.

If your sunburn covers a large area, try a cool bath in plain water. Adding a cup of white vinegar or a generous handful of baking soda to the bathwater may give you additional relief. Colloidal oatmeal in the bath can be very soothing. Purchase Aveeno brand colloidal oatmeal at the drugstore or make your own by grinding ordinary rolled oats in a food processor until they are a fine powder. Put one cup into a tub of cool water and soak for twenty minutes or so.

The discomfort of your sunburn should be a reminder of the value of sunscreen lotions. To avoid burning, use a sunscreen with an SPF (sun protection factor) of at least 15. And remember that you can get a sunburn in the winter, too.

Wear sunscreen if you are active outdoors when there is snow or ice on the ground.

❖ Tooth Care

Your first defense against cavities, gum disease, and other dental ailments is daily brushing and flossing, along with a visit to your dentist twice a year for a checkup and professional cleaning. Your second defense is your diet.

Studies have shown that certain foods can help keep your teeth and gums healthy. Some cheeses, such as blue, Brie, Cheddar, Gouda, mozzarella, Monterey Jack, and Swiss, seem to form a protective barrier on the teeth that helps inhibit the production of cavities. On the other hand, crackers, bread, and other foods that are sticky and cling to your teeth after you eat them lead to cavities. The old custom of ending a meal with a piece of cheese, as it turns out, may be a good idea. Another good idea may be eating your salad last. Fibrous foods such as celery, lettuce, and other raw vegetables help clean your teeth. If you can't brush your teeth or eat salad or cheese after eating especially sticky or sugary foods, even rinsing your mouth well with water can help.

Although a bewildering array of toothpastes are continually advertised, dentists agree that any one that has fluoride is a good choice. This mineral helps strengthen the protective enamel of your teeth throughout your life and is routinely added to drinking water in most communities. The beneficial effects of fluoride can be seen in today's sharply lower cavity rates for young children—nearly half have no cavities in their permanent teeth. But if you choose a natural toothpaste that does not contain fluoride, you lose the beneficial effects. Similarly, if you drink only pure bottled water, you will not get any protective fluoride.

See also Bad Breath; Gum Diseases.

❖ Ulcerative Colitis

Abdominal pain and bloody diarrhea are the main symptoms of ulcerative colitis, a disease that causes ulceration and inflammation of the inner lining of the large intestine and rectum. Other symptoms include fatigue, weight loss, loss of appetite, and rectal bleeding. Some 250,000 Americans have ulcerative colitis. It occurs mostly in young people ages fifteen to forty, although older people sometimes develop the disease, too. Ulcerative colitis is usually a chronic, lifelong disease, but most patients manage to lead normal, productive lives and often have long symptom-free periods.

The cause of ulcerative colitis is unknown, and there is no cure. In very severe cases, doctors resort to surgery to remove part or all of the colon. Fortunately, many patients find that taking their medicine and paying careful attention to diet helps control their symptoms. Because every patient has different responses to particular foods, the simplest approach is to simply keep a record of what you eat and note which foods seem to upset you. In some cases, highly seasoned or high-fiber foods may worsen your symptoms. In many cases, avoiding milk and milk products helps quite a bit, perhaps because lactose intolerance is also a problem.

On the whole, it is very important for ulcerative colitis patients to get good nutrition to compensate for their reduced appetites, poor absorption of nutrients through the intestines, and frequent diarrhea. You may find that eating several small meals a day instead of three larger ones can help. Eating nutritious snacks when you are hungry between meals is also helpful. The severe diarrhea of ulcerative colitis can lead to imbalances in your body's fluids. If you are having diarrhea, your doctor will probably recommend that you drink lots of clear fluids and eat soft, bland foods. You may need to take a prescription medicine to control your diarrhea and other symptoms. These medications are usually very effective.

Cigarette smoking can actually have a protective effect against ulcerative colitis. Studies show that the risk of ulcerative colitis in smokers is reduced by 50 percent or more. On the other hand, smokers are twice as likely to develop Crohn's disease, another form of irritable bowel disease. Since ulcerative colitis may be the only example of a beneficial effect from smoking, and is offset by so many other health problems, it's not a good reason to start or continue smoking.

See also Crohn's Disease; Irritable Bowel Syndrome; Lactose Intolerance.

❖ Ulcers

Any number of myths surround the surprisingly common problem of ulcers. Here are a few: hard-driving, harried executive types are more likely to get ulcers; stress causes ulcers; and drinking milk is good for ulcers. Here's the truth: Ulcers can affect anyone; in many if not most cases, they are caused by a bacteria; and drinking milk can make them worse.

An ulcer is a craterlike sore on the lining of the digestive tract. Most ulcers occur in the duodenum, the first part of your small intestine. Gastric ulcers occur in the stomach. Sometimes ulcers occur in the esophagus, the tube that leads from your mouth to your stomach. Ulcers affect some nineteen million Americans at least once in their lifetime. They most commonly first appear in people between the ages of thirty and fifty.

Ulcers are often caused by damage to the membranes that line your digestive tract. Acid and other fluids from your stomach can then burn the lining and cause a sore. Some anti-inflammatory drugs, such as aspirin, ibuprofen, and prescription drugs for arthritis, can damage the stomach lining and cause ulcers. If you smoke, you are more likely to get ulcers.

Ulcer symptoms are hard to miss because they are so uncomfortable. The most common symptom is a gnawing or burning pain in the abdomen between the lower end of the breastbone and the navel. The pain often occurs between meals and in the early hours of the morning. It may last for a few minutes to a few hours and is often temporarily relieved by eating or taking an antacid. Other ulcer symptoms include nausea, vomiting, and appetite loss.

Doctors used to treat ulcers by prescribing a bland diet and urging patients to drink milk or cream. Today, the usual treatment is a normal diet combined with antibiotics and drugs that reduce the production of stomach acid; nonprescription liquid antacids are also often recommended. No food, no matter how spicy, is known to cause ulcers, although some patients find that a bland diet is easier to tolerate during a flare-up of ulcer symptoms. Others find that fatty or acidic foods aggravate their symptoms. Once recommended for ulcers, milk can actually make them worse because the calcium in it signals your stomach to make more acid. Although no beverage is known to cause ulcers, carbonated beverages can make your symptoms worse. Some patients report that drinking fresh cabbage juice helps their symptoms, despite a lack of scientific basis for this. Drinking alcohol will worsen your ulcer and keep it from healing as quickly. If you drink alcohol, do so in moderation and never on an empty stomach. Caffeine can also slow down the healing process, so avoid coffee (or switch to decaf), tea, and other beverages with caffeine. Eating small, frequent meals when you're having ulcer pain may also help. If your ulcer is caused by prescription drugs, speak to your doctor about cutting back to the minimum dosage and taking the drugs with meals. Over-the-counter antacid liquids may also help deal with drug-induced ulcers, but discuss this with your doctor first.

See also Heartburn; Hiatus Hernia.

❖ Urinary Tract Infections

Every year, some five million people visit their doctors because of a urinary tract infection (UTI). Women are especially prone to them—it is estimated that up to 20 percent of all women develop a UTI sometime in their lives.

The most common symptom of a urinary tract infection is a frequent urge to urinate and a painful, burning sensation during urination. Despite the urge to urinate, you might pass only a small amount of urine, and the urine itself may have a bad odor and appear milky, cloudy, or even have a reddish tinge of blood. Women often experience pain or uncomfortable pressure above the pubic bone. In general, you might feel tired and ill. Children with UTIs often have no symptoms aside from increased urination or they might have symptoms that are confused with those of other illnesses.

Urinary tract infections are usually caused by a bacteria found in the colon, but UTIs can also be caused by the same microorganism that causes the sexually transmitted disease chlamydia. If the bacteria settles in the urethra, the tube that carries urine from the bladder out of the body, urethritis is the result. If the bacteria enters the bladder, cystitis is the result.

Some people are more prone to urinary tract infections than others. Women get them more than men because they have a shorter urethra, so bacteria have a shorter distance to travel to enter the bladder. UTIs are unusual in men. When they do occur, they are usually the result of a kidney stone or an enlarged prostate gland. People with diabetes are also more prone to UTIs because the high levels of sugar in their urine are a fertile breeding ground for bacteria.

If you have a urinary tract infection, your doctor can diagnose it by looking at a sample of your urine. The usual treatment is antibiotics, which often clear up the worst symptoms within a day or two. It's important to finish taking your medicine to avoid recurring infections and to keep from developing a kidney infection. In addition, there are some dietary and self-help steps you can take to relieve symptoms and help prevent a recurrence.

Many women find that they can relieve the pain of a UTI with a warm bath or heating pad. Drinking lots of fluids helps by flushing bacteria out of the urinary tract, but avoid caffeine (especially coffee) and alcohol. Try to drink six to eight glasses of liquid a day, and make one or two of those glasses cranberry or blueberry juice. Compounds in these juices have been shown to help prevent UTI recurrences by keeping bacteria from sticking to the walls of the bladder.

About four out of five women who have a UTI develop another one within eighteen months. To help prevent a recurrence, drink lots of fluids as discussed above. Don't put off urinating when you feel the need, and try to empty your bladder completely each time. Wipe from front to back to prevent bacteria from entering the vagina or urethra. Always urinate shortly before and after sexual intercourse. Avoid using feminine hygiene sprays and scented douches. If you use a diaphragm and get urinary tract infections often, discuss alternative methods of birth control with your doctor.

See also Chlamydia; Vaginitis.

❖ Vaginitis

Vaginitis is a general term for any inflammation of the vagina. The cause is often a yeast infection (candidiasis) or a bacterial infection. The usual culprits in bacterial infections are two organisms: *Gardnerella vaginalis,* which causes bacterial vaginosis, and *Trichomonas vaginalis,* which causes trichomoniasis. (See the section on Yeast Infections for more information about candidiasis.) Some cases of vaginitis are caused by an irritant such as laundry soap or feminine hygiene products. If you have diabetes, you are more likely to get vaginitis. Good hygiene and careful attention to your blood sugar levels can help keep the problem under control.

The signs of bacterial vaginosis include a white, gray, or yellowish vaginal discharge, a fishy odor in the genital area, itching, and a slight redness or swelling of the vagina and vulva. Trichomoniasis causes a watery, yellowish, greenish, bubbly discharge, an unpleasant odor, and pain and itching when urinating. You are most likely to have symptoms after your period. Irritant vaginitis usually causes itching, redness, and a yellowish or white discharge. Bacterial ailments are usually treated with antibiotic pills or a vaginal cream. Don't use yogurt for a bacterial infection—it will make it worse. Some women find that the symptoms of itchiness are relieved by soaking in a warm bath that has a cup of white vinegar added.

Irritant vaginitis has many possible sources: laundry detergent, fabric softeners, feminine hygiene products (such as deodorants or douches), bubble baths, colored toilet paper, scented tampons, latex from condoms or diaphragms, spermicides, or physical irritation (from bike riding, for example). Try different brands of laundry products and avoid putting anything scented or colored near your genitals. Most doctors suggest avoiding feminine hygiene products—they're rarely necessary, and they can cause irritation. If your birth control method is the problem, discuss alternatives with your doctor.

In general, you can reduce the risk of vaginitis and help prevent recurrences by keeping your genital area clean and dry. Wear all-cotton underpants during the day, and skip underpants altogether at night. Avoid wearing tight trousers, leggings, panty hose, bathing suits, leotards, biking shorts, and other tightly fitting apparel for long periods of time. Whenever possible, wear loose clothing made from natural fabrics. Stay out of hot tubs—the shared warm water is a perfect medium for passing germs around. If you have vaginitis, use a condom during intercourse to avoid passing infection to your partner.

See also Chlamydia; Herpes; Urinary Tract Infections; Yeast Infections.

❖ Varicose Veins

The veins have one-way valves in them to keep the blood flowing in one direction. Sometimes, often as a result of standing a lot, the valves don't work well and let blood flow backward. The result is varicose veins—twisted, swollen veins, usually in the legs at the back of the calf or up the inside of your leg.

Varicose veins are often tender to the touch; the skin above the swollen vein may be itchy. Your whole leg may ache and your feet may become swollen; standing or walking for even a short period may make both legs feel sore and tired. In severe cases, varicose veins can lead to a skin ulcer above the vein. A more worrisome complication is the possibility of the vein rupturing or of blood clots forming. In many cases, severe varicose veins can be treated in the doctor's office by sclerotherapy. This involves injecting a solution into the vein that causes the vessel to be absorbed by the body. In some cases, you will need a surgical procedure to remove the vein. In either case, other veins take over the job of circulating the blood.

Some self-help techniques can relieve the discomfort of varicose veins. Most doctors recommend staying off your feet as much as possible, wearing support stockings, and keeping your legs elevated, especially at night. Try raising up the foot of your bed six inches with bricks or wooden blocks.

Diet can also have an effect on your varicose veins. If you keep your weight at normal levels, you are less likely to develop them, since you will not be putting extra pressure on your legs. If you eat a high-fiber diet, you will avoid constipation. Straining during bowel movements puts extra pressure on the veins in your rectum and your legs.

Those spidery webs of blood vessels that appear on your thighs are venous telangiectasia, as the condition is formally called, and not varicose veins. This is more of a cosmetic problem than a medical one. Elevating your legs and eating a high-fiber diet can help.

❖ Yeast Infections

Vaginal yeast infections (candidiasis) are so common that three out of four women will experience one in their lifetime. The symptoms are fairly easy to recognize: moderate to intense itching, an odorless white discharge that resembles cottage cheese, redness and swelling in the vaginal area, vaginal soreness, and a burning sensation, especially during intercourse.

Yeast infections are usually caused by a fungus called *Candida albicans*. This organism is found normally in the vagina, but under certain conditions it can start to multiply rapidly, resulting in a yeast infection. Some of the causes of this include normal hormonal changes, antibiotics, douching, pregnancy, diabetes, certain kinds of birth control pills and spermicides, and being hot and sweaty for long periods. Some unfortunate women seem to get yeast infections for no particular reason at all.

If you've never had a yeast infection before, see your doctor for a firm diagnosis. Yeast infections usually respond well to treatment with nonprescription antifungal medicines containing either clotrimazole or miconazole nitrate.

If you get frequent yeast infections, there are some practical steps you can take to avoid recurrences. Wear all-cotton underpants during the day, and skip underpants altogether at night.

Avoid wearing tight trousers, panty hose, leggings, bathing suits, leotards, biking shorts, and other tightly fitting apparel for long periods. Whenever possible, wear loose clothing made from natural fabrics. Also avoid feminine hygiene products such as deodorants or douches, after-bath powder containing talc or cornstarch, bubble baths, colored toilet paper, and scented tampons. If you suspect that your birth control method is causing the problem, discuss alternatives with your doctor.

There is some evidence that women who eat a lot of sugar have more yeast infections, so try cutting back on sweets if yeast infections are a problem for you. A preventive measure that seems to work for many women is eating a cup of plain, live-culture yogurt every day. Most supermarket yogurt does not contain live acidophilus bacteria—try your health food store instead. Do not put yogurt in your vagina, however. Some women are helped by eliminating or limiting foods that contain yeast or mold: bread, baked goods, cheese, beer, wine, pickles, fermented foods, and mushrooms. Others find that restricting milk and milk products helps.

See also Vaginitis.

Healing
Foods

❖ Alfalfa

Alfalfa is a member of the legume (bean) family. Low in calories and low in fat, it's high in the B vitamins, vitamin C, vitamin K, carotene, chlorophyll, and eight essential enzymes. Alfalfa is also a good source of biotin, calcium, iron, and protein. For years, alfalfa sprouts were only sold in health food stores, but now they're in the produce section of most supermarkets. They're even relatively easy to grow at home in window boxes. Alfalfa sprouts can be used in salads, in sandwiches (try them with a melted cheese sandwich), atop pizza, and even on the side at dinner, along with your other favorite vegetables. In juice form, alfalfa is a tasty way to get a good portion of your daily vitamins and minerals.

Alfalfa is a great health food for most people, but avoid it if you have the autoimmune disorder lupus. The amino acid L-canavanine in the alfalfa can make lupus symptoms worse.

❖ Almonds

Although terrifically high in fat (13 grams of fat per ounce), almonds are rich in monounsaturated fatty acids and high in vitamin E. What's more, almonds are one of the best nondairy sources of calcium: 1 ounce gives you about 10 percent of the recommended daily allowance. Almonds are also a good source of riboflavin and the trace mineral boron. But calorie counters beware: just 1/2 cup packs a whopping 400 calories.

Cook's Note
Almonds can be used whole, slivered, sliced, or ground into a paste. Sometimes almonds require blanching to remove their papery skins. To blanch almonds, cover then with boiling water and let them soak for about five minutes. Drain well, then rub the skins off with your fingers. One pound of almonds (in their shells) yields about 1 1/4 cups.

❖ Amaranth

A tiny, poppy seed–sized grain that was once a staple food of the Aztecs, amaranth is loaded with protein and calcium. Its mild, nutty flavor cooks up to make a great hot breakfast cereal; for a change of pace, serve it as you would rice at dinnertime. This low-calorie, low-fat, high-fiber grain is delicious toasted; you can add it to pancake, muffin, and cake batters or use it to enliven salads and soups. Amaranth is high in vitamins and minerals, especially calcium—1/2 cup contains as much calcium as a glass of milk, but has only sixteen calories. Amaranth is also very high in lysine, one of the essential amino acids. The high-quality protein of this grain makes it a good choice for vegetarians or occasional meatless eating.

❖ Apples

The original health food, apples are low in sodium and high in fiber. Checking in at only 81 calories each, they have just a single gram of fat and no cholesterol. Apples contain potassium, a mineral that helps regulate the body's fluid balance and neuromuscular activity, and they are a good source of the trace mineral boron, which is needed for healthy bones. One medium-sized apple provides about a third of your daily boron requirement. An average-sized apple has less sodium than a stalk of celery, a carrot, or a glass of ordinary tap water and has more fiber than a bowl of most popular cereals, including oatmeal.

Eating an apple a day (with the skin) is one of the simplest, cheapest, and most enjoyable ways to prevent constipation. More than 80 percent of the fiber in an apple is water-soluble pectin, the type of fiber credited with helping to lower blood cholesterol levels. Pectin can also help relieve diarrhea symptoms. In fact, many doctors suggest eating applesauce or grated apples if you're having a bout of intestinal flu. On the other hand, the high levels of pectin in apple juice can give some people, especially children, mild diarrhea. One other minor drawback: apples can produce gas in some people. You don't have to skip the benefits of this delicious, easy-to-find fruit because of that, though. Try eating just half an apple instead. The sweet taste and crispness of a fresh apple are very satisfying for dieters. Try eating an apple half an hour before mealtime—you could find that you naturally eat less without feeling hungry or deprived.

In the United States, there are more than two dozen apple varieties available virtually year round. Choose fresh, firm, well-colored apples. Store them in a ventilated plastic bag or hydrator drawer in the refrigerator to prevent absorbing other food flavors. And in case you're wondering about the white film you sometimes see on apples, it's a natural wax that is reapplied after the harvest (the natural wax is washed off) to retain freshness and crispness. The wax is approved by the U.S. Food and Drug Administration. Some of the most popular apple varieties are listed below:

McIntosh. Used for cooking and eating, its flavor ranges from tart to slightly sweet.

Granny Smith. The usual choice for pies, this green, tart, and crunchy apple is ideal for most cooking and baking.

Delicious (red or golden). Perhaps the most popular apples. Sweet and delicious eaten out of hand, they're also good in salads.

Rome Beauty. Green-yellow apples with tinges of red. They keep well and are also good for baking.

Cortland. Crisp, tart, great in applesauce, this apple is a hybrid of the McIntosh.

Empire. Another McIntosh hybrid, this all-purpose fruit is used for both eating and cooking.

Northern Pippin. Crisp, tart, and yellow-green in color, this is a very good cooking apple.

Jonathan. Juicy red cooking apples, they're often used in making pies and tarts.

Cook's Note

Three medium-sized apples equal approximately 1 pound, which is equivalent to about 3 cups peeled, sliced, or diced fruit.

❖ Apricots

One of the stone fruits (along with cherries, nectarines, peaches, and plums), apricots have, at their best, a rich, sweet, peachlike flavor with hints of wine and lemon. Nutritionally, apricots are abundant in vitamin A. As all the orange-colored fruits and vegetables do, apricots contain large amounts of beta carotene, an antioxidant substance that may help prevent cancer. Three small fresh apricots (which is one serving by USDA standards) have more than 50 percent of the RDA for beta carotene, all for a mere 50 calories and no fat. (Even canned apricots in heavy syrup are low in calories—1/2 cup has just 105 calories.) Apricots are also good sources of potassium, magnesium, and iron.

Apricots are at their freshness peak from June through August, although they are also delicious—and have a more intense flavor—dried. Sulfur dioxide is often used to preserve dried apricots. While most people have no problem with this, some are allergic to sulfites, and sulfites can also trigger migraine headaches. Sulfite-free dried fruit is readily available at natural food stores.

Apricot pits contain enough cyanide to be potentially dangerous. Don't swallow or suck on the pits.

Cook's Note

To plump dried apricots, soak them in hot water for about ten minutes, then drain them before using them in a recipe. To peel fresh apricots, drop them in boiling water for about thirty seconds, rinse in cold water, and peel. Peeled fruit will discolor when exposed to the air, so brush the surface with a little lemon juice to keep the color intact.

❖ Artichokes

Did you know that when you eat an artichoke, you're actually eating a flower bud? If allowed to flower, blossoms measure up to seven inches in diameter and are a beautiful violet blue. Artichokes are low in calories (about 30 each), high in fiber (nearly 2 grams each), and are a good natural source of folic acid. (Women who are of childbearing age are urged to consume 400 micrograms of folic acid daily to prevent neural tube defects in their babies.) Artichokes are also high in calcium, phosphorus, potassium, magnesium, B vitamins, and sodium. If you need to limit your sodium intake, avoid artichokes. Although artichokes are traditionally recommended for liver and gallbladder ailments, there is little evidence that they have any useful effect. It's possible that artichokes could help lower your blood cholesterol—some studies suggest that artichoke extracts might have a beneficial effect.

The globe artichoke is a member of the thistle family, and is at its peak in March, April, and May. When available in colder months, the chokes often have a purple tinge, which indicates frostbite, but there is no loss of flavor or texture. The edible flower bud is enclosed by green, leaflike scales or bracts. Both the bracts and flower base (or heart) are edible. The best artichokes have tight, thick bracts and a vibrant green color.

Cook's Note

Store artichokes in a plastic bag in the refrigerator for up to seven days. Artichokes can be steamed, boiled, microwaved, or sautéed. For example, steam them for about thirty minutes, or until a leaf pulls out easily and the heart is tender when pierced with the tip of a knife. Don't use an aluminum, iron, or carbon steel pot, as these metals may discolor the artichokes and impart a bitter flavor to them. Plan on one medium-sized artichoke per person.

❖ Asparagus

A favorite food of the ancient Egyptians and Greeks, asparagus are low in calories (just 23 calories per 1/2 cup) and high in protein. An excellent source of iron, vitamin A, and vitamin C, that same 1/2 cup of asparagus can also provide you with about 25 percent of your RDA for folic acid. Another compound found in asparagus, the antioxidant glutathione, could help protect you against cancer. A member of the lily family, asparagus is also a natural diuretic, which helps prevent water retention. After eating asparagus, many people notice a strong odor in their urine. This is due to the excretion of an amino acid called asparagine. This is in no way detrimental and the effect is only temporary.

Cook's Note

Look for asparagus in its peak season, April through May. Select spears that are firm, crisp, and well rounded. Tips should be closed and free from damage. Try to select uniform spears for ease of cooking. Allow about 1/3 pound per serving. You can store asparagus up to four days in perforated plastic bags in the refrigerator. Keep the bases wrapped in moist paper toweling for maximum freshness. Steam fresh asparagus in a covered skillet over medium heat for five to ten minutes, depending on the thickness of the stalks. Asparagus should be a bright green when cooked.

❖ Avocado

If avocados make you think of California cuisine, you're not far off the mark: 60 percent of all avocados are consumed in California, and it's one of the top twenty best-selling fruits in the United States. Half an avocado gives you about 160 calories, and a hefty portion of fat: 13.7 grams. But the news isn't as grim as it sounds: of the total fat, 9.7 grams (over 80 percent) consists of monounsaturated fatty acids—the same healthful fatty acid that's found in olive oil. Avocados are also surprisingly high in fiber—half a medium-sized avocado has 4 grams.

Avocados are a nutrient-dense fruit. They pack in a significant amount of vitamin A: well over 500 IUs—more than any other fruit, including apples—as well as over 500 milligrams of potassium. Glutathione, a powerful antioxidant, is also found in avocados.

Cook's Note

Avocados are available year round, and most supermarkets carry California (usually Hass variety) or Florida (Fuerte) avocados. The Hass variety has dark, bumpy skin and is richer in taste, calories, and fat than the Fuerte avocados. When choosing avocados, look for firm, unblemished fruit. To ripen, place them in a paper bag or fruit basket near other fruit. The ripeness test: the flesh should yield to gentle pressure from your fingers. Slice avocados in half, cutting the flesh around the pit. Twist the halves in opposite directions to separate. Despite what some people say, placing an avocado pit in guacamole (a spicy Mexican dip made from avocados) won't keep the guacamole from turning brown. Instead, sprinkle the top of the guacamole with lemon juice and cover the bowl tightly with plastic wrap.

❖ Bananas

Bananas come in several varieties in addition to the one that we know best: yellow, smooth-skinned, and available year round in the United States. Look for Red Jamaican, plantains, and other varieties in large supermarkets and ethnic markets. The average yellow banana, at a mere 100 calories and no fat, contains 450 milligrams of potassium as well as 25 percent of the RDA for Vitamin B_6 and 15 percent of the RDA for vitamin C.

Many doctors suggest eating bananas if you have diarrhea. They're easy to digest, nutritious, and won't irritate your bowels further. The pectin in the bananas helps relieve diarrhea symptoms, and it may also help protect you against colon cancer. Eating bananas often relieves the symptoms of indigestion with nausea and could help heal gastric ulcers. Because bananas are fairly bland and easy to mash, they go down easily if you have a sore throat or trouble swallowing.

Cook's Note

Bananas are picked unripe. They turn yellow with some brown freckling as they ripen at room temperature. You can ripen bananas overnight by placing them in a brown paper bag. (A good way to ripen other fruit is to put it into a brown paper bag with a banana.) If you're not concerned about the skin color, you can refrigerate ripe bananas: the skin will blacken, but the fruit will remain white for two to three days. Try it—a refrigerated banana tastes a little like banana ice cream without the calories.

❖ Barley

One of the oldest cultivated grains, barley is an excellent source of soluble fiber. It is often recommended as food to help lower blood cholesterol levels, especially the LDLs (low-density lipoproteins, or "bad" cholesterol). Barley is a good dietary source of chromium, a mineral that helps your body regulate its use of insulin. (Many doctors now suggest that patients with Type II diabetes eat barley often.) Of course, as a vegetable food, barley has no cholesterol itself and is very low in fat: just 1 gram in 3 ounces of uncooked barley. There are only 120 calories in 1/2 cup of cooked barley. It is very low in gluten, making it a good choice for people with celiac disease and wheat allergies. In general, barley makes a nice change of pace from rice as a side dish or in soups and casseroles. The mild flavor and slightly chewy texture blend well with sauces and gravies.

Cook's Note

Barley is commonly available in three forms: pearl, whole hulled, and groats. The pearl variety is the barley grain stripped of husks and germ (interestingly, the cholesterol-fighting substances in barley are not in the husk, so you still get that benefit). It is white, cooks rather quickly, and is available in coarse, medium, and fine textures. The quick-cooking version is essentially pearl barley that has been presteamed; the grains are flattened, but the taste is the same. Pearl barley cooks in forty-five to sixty minutes. Quick-cooking barley cooks in ten to fifteen minutes. Whole hulled barley, available in health food stores, has a gritty texture, brown color, and high fiber content, because the outer coating or hull is left on. Use this kind in soups and stews. A third variety, barley groats, is the least processed, but in this form the grain takes a long time to cook. You can really only use barley groats in slow-cooked soups or as a porridge.

❖ Beans

They're protein-rich, full of fiber, low in fat, and low in cholesterol, so if you haven't been eating beans, you should start adding them to your diet. Besides being rich in nutrients, they're flavorful, inexpensive, and easy to prepare. In fact, beans are so nutritious and full of protein that they're included in both the vegetable and protein groups in the USDA's food pyramid. Beans give you iron, potassium, calcium, zinc, magnesium, phosphorus, and other essential minerals. They are also a great natural source of the B-complex vitamins. And because they're a complex carbohydrate and digest more slowly than most other carbohydrate foods, they satisfy hunger longer. If you're dieting, beans are a boon. For the same number of calories, you can eat between two and four times the amount of beans as meat or cheese, and only about 5 percent of those calories will come from fat. Many diabetics find that adding beans to their diet helps them better control their blood sugar levels, since digesting the beans releases glucose slowly and steadily instead of in spurts.

Beans are famous (or infamous) for producing gas. The reason for this is that the bean skins contain indigestible sugars; when the beans enter your lower intestine, the bacteria that are normally there feast on the sugars; producing gas as a by-product. There are some useful steps you can take to reduce the gas level. If you're soaking your own dried beans, use three cups of water for every cup of beans. Drain the beans and change the water at least twice during the twenty-four-hour soaking period. Drain the beans and rinse them well before using. If you're using convenient canned beans, drain them and rinse them well before using. Finally, be sure to cook the beans thoroughly. Don't add baking soda to the beans—it doesn't cut the gas and it toughens the beans. You could try a commercial product called Beano. It contains an enzyme that helps you digest the sugars before they reach the lower intestine.

Beans, also called legumes, are the seeds of any plant that has pods. Technically speaking, then, peanuts are legumes. There are thousands of bean varieties, but only about twenty-five or so are commonly used in cooking. Below is a quick rundown of twelve of the most popular:

Adzuki beans. These small, red beans used widely in Asian cooking have a mild, sweet taste.

Baby limas. Mild-flavored, they are usually served as a vegetable or in casseroles.

Black beans. Small black beans are also known as turtle beans and are a staple of Central and South American cooking.

Broad beans (fava beans). These large, flat beans range in color from white to brown. Most recipes call for the skins to be removed—they slip off easily.

Cannellini beans. These white, kidney-shaped beans are popular in Italian cooking.

Garbanzos (chickpeas). Round and yellow gold in color, these beans have a nutlike flavor. Ideal in salads and appetizers, they are often used in Italian, Middle Eastern, and Indian cooking.

Great northern. These medium-sized white beans are often used in soups.

Kidney. Red and kidney-shaped, these are among the most popular beans. Use them in chili, bean salads, and in pasta dishes.

Large lima. This shell bean has a rich, buttery flavor. Serve it as a side vegetable.

Navy. Small white beans, so called because they were once a staple in navy mess halls, are the traditional bean for navy bean soup and Boston baked beans.

Pinto. These pink beans dotted with specks of red are traditionally used to make Mexican refried beans.

Soybeans. These cream-colored beans have a strong flavor, are fairly high in fat, and take a long time to cook. They are usually used in other forms such as soy milk, tofu (bean curd), soy flour, and textured vegetable protein.

See also individual beans.

❖ Bean Sprouts

Traditional Chinese bean sprouts are the sprouts of mung beans. Available year round in most supermarkets, they are very low in calories, high in vitamin C, and give you 1.6 grams of fiber per cup. Crisp and white, they can be used fresh or blanched for thirty seconds to remove the raw taste. (If you blanch them, refresh them in ice water and drain well before using.) Bean sprouts add nutrition and crunch to salads and sandwiches, and they're great in stir-fries. Bean sprouts keep up to four days in the refrigerator.

❖ Bee Pollen

The golden dust gathered by bees from the stamen of flowers, bee pollen has enjoyed some sensational press, mostly due to its use by Great Britain's royal family. Sensational stories aside, some natural medicine practitioners and nutritionists claim that bee pollen can enhance your vitality. Bee pollen contains 185 nutrients (including twenty-two amino acids), a full array of vitamins (including a good amount of vitamin B_{12}), and many minerals such as calcium, iron, and potassium. It's possible that a daily spoonful or two could give you the vitamins and minerals you need just as well as a vitamin tablet. Proponents of bee pollen claim that it fights fatigue, depression, and has an antimicrobial effect. Some people who are allergic to pollen may be allergic to bee pollen, however. Stop taking it if you develop a rash, wheeze, get hives, or have any other related symptoms.

❖ Beets

A vegetable with both edible roots and leaves, beets are high in vitamins A and C and contain calcium and iron as well. Fresh or canned, beets check in with only 53 calories for a 1-cup serving. Beets are high in sodium, however; they have about 400 milligrams per cup. Beet fiber has been reported to have a positive effect on lowering cholesterol levels and improving bowel function. Beets are the main ingredient of an eastern European favorite, borscht, a thick red soup served either hot or cold.

Cook's Note

Choose firm beets less than two inches in diameter. You can store the roots in the refrigerator for about a week. Cook beets before peeling them. This helps retain their color as they cook; the skins will come off easily if you plunge the beets into cold water after cooking.

❖ Beet Greens

In Roman times, beets were grown so that their tops could be cut off and eaten as a vegetable. Beet greens are dark green with red veins. The greens are an excellent source of calcium, vitamin A, and folic acid (folate), an essential B vitamin.

Cook's Note

The greens should be fresh looking, with no damaged, yellowed, or wilted leaves. To store, trim off the greens, then wash them thoroughly, and store them separately in plastic bags lined with paper toweling. The greens will keep for about three days.

❖ Berries

Anyone who's ever been on diet or is just watching calories has been grateful for berries: they're deliciously sweet *and* low in calories. Raspberries, for example, are intensely sweet but have just 100 calories per cup. They also have a good amount of vitamin C and potassium, and 3.3 grams of dietary fiber. Nutritionally, all berries are good sources of B vitamins, vitamin C, and water-soluble fiber.

The vivid colors of berries come from plant pigments called flavonoids. Research suggests that flavonoids protect your cells against free radical damage. Berries, especially raspberries, blackberries, and strawberries, are good sources of a compound called ellagic acid, which is believed to have cancer-preventing properties. Fragile berries such as raspberries, loganberries, boysenberries, dewberries, and blackberries are all related and have similar nutritional properties. Other berries include gooseberries and cranberries, which are small, firm, and very tart; they need to be cooked and sweetened to be palatable.

Cook's Note

All berries are picked ripe and have a short shelf life. Steer clear of berries in packaging that has become wet or stained by berry juice since moisture makes berries deteriorate rapidly. Do not wash berries before storing. To freeze berries, arrange them in a single layer on a tray and freeze for about two hours. Then pour the berries into a resealable plastic bag, press out the air, and seal. Use within two months for best flavor. Strawberries should always have a deep red color; avoid greenish ones or ones with white near the tops, as strawberries do not ripen off the vine. Always wash strawberries with their caps on to avoid soaking the hull.

See also Blueberries; Cranberries.

❖ Bitter Melon (Balsam Pear)

A tropical fruit, bitter melon resembles a green cucumber with large, warty lumps on its surface. Look for it in Asian grocery stores. Bitter melon is grown in Asia, South America, and Africa, and as the name suggests, it is quite bitter. In India and elsewhere, bitter melon is used as a traditional treatment for diabetes. There may be some scientific basis for this: unripe bitter melon does contain compounds that can help lower blood sugar levels in diabetics. Some evidence also suggests that bitter melon compounds could be effective for fighting leukemia.

❖ Black-Eyed Peas

These creamy-colored beans have a black "eye" or dot in the center and cook up with an earthy flavor. Like other beans, black-eyed peas (also called cowpeas) are rich in protein and fiber and low in fat and cholesterol. They're also one of the best dietary sources of folic acid. One 3 1/2-ounce serving has 440 micrograms—twice the RDA for a woman. Unlike most beans, black-eyed peas also contain vitamin A.

Cook's Note
In the South, black-eyed peas are traditionally served on New Year's Day to bring good luck in the coming year in hoppin' John, a dish that features rice, peas, and salt pork. Black-eyed peas have a thin skin and are one of the few beans that can be cooked without presoaking.

❖ Blueberries

The rich, sweet flavor of blueberries made them a favorite food of Native Americans. The Indians of the Pacific Northwest, for example, preserved blueberries by smoking them and used them as a seasoning in soups and with meats. The

Indians of the Northeast mixed sun-dried blueberries with cornmeal, and blueberries were on the menu at the first Thanksgiving. Although blueberries grow wild across North America, most cultivated blueberries are grown in Maine, Michigan, New Jersey, Quebec, and Nova Scotia; blueberries are also commercially grown in North Carolina and the Pacific Northwest region.

Cultivated blueberries contain a wide range of nutrients. They are naturally high in vitamin C and fiber, have very little fat, and are very low in sodium. A cup of fresh blueberries has 80 calories, 1 gram of protein, 17 grams of carbohydrate, and 4 grams of dietary fiber. That same cup would provide 15 percent of the RDA for vitamin C and 105 milligrams of potassium. The fiber in blueberries consists largely of pectin. This soluble fiber may help protect against colon cancer and can help lower cholesterol levels.

Blueberries are one of the few foods that are naturally blue in color. Most of the blue fruits, including other berries and grapes, contain large amounts of a complex organic compound called anthocyanoside. In concentrated form, this compound has been shown to help slow vision loss due to macular degeneration.

Botanically speaking, blueberries and cranberries are closely related. Cranberry juice has been shown to help prevent bladder infections in women, and blueberries can have the same effect. The reason is that both berries contain a substance that blocks infection-causing bacteria from adhering to the bladder.

Cook's Note

Blueberries are a good snack choice for people on weight-loss or low-sodium diets. Naturally sweet but still low in calories, they are satisfying on their own or added to hot or cold cereal, yogurt, and fruit salads. Fresh berries should have crisp, unblemished outer skins. Save frozen blueberries to use in baking as an addition to muffins and pound cakes, or add them to pancake and waffle batters.

❖ Bok Choy (Chinese Cabbage)

For a healthy dose of beta carotene, include bok choy—a favorite Chinese vegetable—in your diet. A cup of this leafy green vegetable contains nearly 100 percent of the RDA for beta carotene, as well as valuable amounts of vitamin C, potassium, and other vitamins and minerals, all for a trifling 15 calories. Bok choy can also help you meet your calcium requirement: 1 cup gives you nearly the same amount as half a glass of milk—about 150 milligrams. Bok choy is a member of the cruciferous family of vegetables, which means it is high in the cancer-fighting antioxidants called indoles.

Cook's Note

Bok choy has long, white stalks and large, dark green leaves. Look for compact bunches with fresh, glossy leaves and unblemished stalks. Bok choy is delicious eaten raw, but it is at its best in traditional Chinese stir-fried dishes.

Bran

Bran is a general term that refers to the fibrous outer husk of seeds and grains, such as wheat, rice, oats, and barley. Because the bran is made of tough fiber, it is often removed by a polishing process. White rice is rice without the bran, and it cooks quickly and has a soft texture. Brown rice is rice that still has its bran, which is why it takes longer to cook and has a chewier texture. Removing the bran, however, also removes some of the healthful fiber and B vitamins from the grain.

Bran is an excellent source of fiber (see the discussion of fiber on page 8 for more information). Adding it to your diet could help prevent constipation, colon cancer, and diverticular disease. Diabetics often benefit from adding bran to their diets, since it can help lower blood sugar levels. Oat bran and wheat bran in particular can help lower blood cholesterol levels.

See also Oats; Wheat Bran.

❖ Brazil Nuts

A high oil content gives these large, cream-colored nut meats a rich taste and a lot of calories. High in thiamine and magnesium, they also contain iron, zinc, and calcium. Brazil nuts are also the richest food source of selenium, a trace mineral your body needs to make the antioxidant enzyme glutathione. (People with low levels of selenium have a higher risk of cancer, heart disease, and fibrocystic breast disease; selenium deficiency is also linked to depression.) One Brazil nut contains about 100 micrograms of selenium, or somewhat more than the recommended dietary allowance. Don't overdo the Brazil nuts—too much selenium is toxic. Because of their high oil content, Brazil nuts go rancid rapidly; buy only as much as you will use within a few days.

See also Nuts.

❖ Brewer's Yeast

Also sometimes called nutritional yeast, brewer's yeast is a brown powder made from the same one-celled organisms that are used to ferment beer. Because it is very high in protein and contains many vitamins (including most of the B vitamins), minerals, and amino acids, brewer's yeast is sometimes used as a food supplement, particularly by athletes. Herbalists and natural medicine practitioners often recommend it as an energy booster. The powder is usually taken in capsules or mixed with juice or water. Despite claims, there is little or no evidence that brewer's yeast helps heart problems, diabetes, eczema, psoriasis, or gout. Neither will it keep fleas or mosquitoes away.

❖ Broccoli

Broccoli is a powerhouse of a vegetable, packed with nutrients, fiber, and antioxidant compounds. A single large stalk (one serving) provides 120 percent of the RDA for vitamin C and 35 percent for vitamin A; that same serving also has about 150 milligrams of calcium, about 600 milligrams of potassium, 200 micrograms of folic acid, virtually no sodium, and a healthy 2 grams of fiber, all for only 50 calories. Broccoli contains chromium, a mineral that helps your body regulate its use of insulin. (Many doctors now suggest that patients with Type II diabetes eat broccoli often.) Boron, a mineral you need in trace amounts to regulate the electrical activity in your brain, is also found in broccoli. Like other cruciferous vegetables (cabbage, kale, brussels sprouts), broccoli contains a number of valuable antioxidant compounds—quercetin, glutathione, and sulforaphane, among others—that have been linked to reduced risk of cancer. Indoles, another compound in broccoli and other cruciferous vegetables, may neutralize the hormones that could activate tumors in estrogen-sensitive areas, particularly the breast. Indoles may also help relieve breast tenderness from fibrocystic breast disease.

Cook's Note

Look for firm stalks with tight green heads; yellowing heads indicate that the broccoli is past its peak. Broccoli lasts for up to four days in the refrigerator in a plastic bag. Remove the outer leaves and cut off the tough ends of the stems for the most even cooking. To get the most from broccoli's nutrients, cook it lightly or eat it raw.

❖ Brussels Sprouts

Brussels sprouts look like miniature cabbages and are indeed members of the cabbage family. As such, this vegetable is dense with nutrients. Like broccoli, brussels sprouts contain cancer-fighting compounds, including indoles and sulforaphane. Brussels sprouts also contain a remarkable amount of fiber: 7.5 grams in a single cup. They're high in vitamin C and contribute significantly to your recommended daily allowance of other vitamins and minerals. One cup of cooked brussels sprouts contains 800 IU of vitamin A, 400 milligrams of potassium, and 110 milligrams of phosphorus.

Cook's Note

Brussels sprouts heads should be bright green and firm. It's best to use them within two days. To cook, remove any loose outer leaves. With a sharp paring knife, cut an X into the bottom stem of each sprout; this helps them cook through more evenly. The key with brussels sprouts is not to overcook them. Their delicate flavor and firm texture turn into a bitter and unpalatable mush when overdone.

❖ Buckwheat (Kasha)

Despite its name, buckwheat is not a type of wheat, and doesn't come from a grass, although it is a type of grain. The small, pyramidal kernels of buckwheat, also known as kasha, are in fact the seeds of a flowering plant. The kernels have a soft brown color and a distinctively nutty flavor. High in fiber and low in both fat and calories, buckwheat is also high in all eight essential amino acids, especially lysine. (If you suffer from herpes or cold sores, lysine could help them clear up faster.) Additionally, buckwheat is gluten-free, which makes it a good grain substitute for people with celiac disease or wheat allergies, since buckwheat is closer to being a complete protein than any other plant food. It can be a valuable protein source for vegetarians.

Cook's Note

Buckwheat groats are available in whole, medium, and fine granulations. The whole grain holds its shape and texture the best, but takes a little longer to cook. All buckwheat granulations will hold their texture best if toasted lightly in a hot skillet before cooking. Buckwheat flour makes deliciously light pancakes. Japanese soba noodles are made from a combination of wheat and buckwheat flours.

❖ Bulgur

A quick-cooking wheat grain that has been parboiled, dried, and crushed, bulgur is a wonderful source of fiber. A tasty alternative to rice, it is nutritious, too. Bulgur is high in protein, phosphorus, calcium, iron, and potassium and rich in B vitamins; it's low in fat, sodium, and calories.

Cook's Note

Bulgur is the grain base of tabbouleh, a popular Middle Eastern salad. It can also substitute for rice in many pilafs. Bulgur is not the same as cracked wheat—bulgur cooks much more quickly. The finer the grind, the quicker it cooks. As a rule of thumb, one cup of uncooked bulgur yields approximately 2 1/2 cups cooked grains. Refrigerate any unused grain in an airtight container.

❖ Cabbage

The American Cancer Society strongly recommends a diet high in cruciferous vegetables, such as cabbage, broccoli, brussels sprouts, and cauliflower. Cabbages and other members of the cabbage family contain valuable antioxidants and other substances that could help prevent cancer. Cabbage is also a rich source of calcium, vitamin C, potassium, and iron. What's more, it's incredibly low in calories: just 17 per cup for raw, shredded cabbage. If you have ulcers, it's possible that drinking fresh cabbage juice will help them heal up faster.

Cook's Note

Cabbages should be firm and heavy for their size. Most varieties keep well for up to two weeks in the refrigerator. Several popular varieties of cabbage are easily found in your supermarket:

Green cabbage. Look for firm, round heads with light green or white leaves.

Red cabbage. This variety has purple-red leaves (which will turn blue if you cook them with an acidic substance, such as citrus juice). The taste is basically the same as green cabbage.

Savoy cabbage. Crinkled, flexible, light green leaves distinguish this cabbage.

Napa cabbage. Look for firm, oblong heads with long, white ribs and light green tips with frills.

Bok choy (Chinese cabbage) This type has long white stalks and large, dark green leaves.

❖ Carob

The sweet, molasseslike flavor of carob is faintly reminiscent of chocolate, although a true chocoholic will find carob a paltry substitute for the real thing. However, when used as a flavoring on its own merit, it's quite pleasant. The fruit pod of the carob tree, carob is also known as locust bean, locust pod, and St. John's bread (because St. John was said to have eaten carob with honey while traveling in the desert). Ounce for ounce, carob is sweeter than chocolate, so if you use it in baking, you may not have to add any additional sugar. Unlike chocolate, carob is caffeine-free, but it contains similar amounts of fat and calories. One ounce of carob chips has 140 calories and 7 grams of fat; an equivalent amount of chocolate has 143 calories and 10 grams of fat.

Cook's Note

In addition to carob chips and carob bars, you can buy carob powder, which can be added to regular flour to create carob flour.

❖ Carrots

Carrots have an abundance of beta carotene and fiber. Beta carotene, the precursor to vitamin A, is one of the most effective antioxidants known. Aside from its protective powers against cancer and heart disease, beta carotene promotes healthy eyes and could protect you against developing cataracts and macular degeneration. Beta carotene can also give your immune system a boost, helping you to fend off infections. A single raw carrot gives you some 11,000 IU of vitamin A (which includes beta carotene), or more than 250 percent of the recommended dietary allowance. And carrots also contain water-soluble fiber, which has been shown to help reduce blood cholesterol levels. One raw carrot has about 1 gram of fiber and only about 40 calories.

Cook's Note

Carrots are delicious and nutritious eaten raw, but cooking them briefly actually makes their nutrients more accessible to your body. Choose bright, crisp carrots with no cracks. If the green tops are still attached, they should look green and fresh, not yellowed or wilted. Carrots should always be peeled or scrubbed before eating. If the tips of the carrot are green-hued, cut them off: it is usually an indication of bitterness. Carrots will keep in the refrigerator for at least two weeks; store them in plastic bags. If you are cooking for confirmed carrot haters, try sneaking the carrots into casseroles, stews, and soups. And nearly everyone loves carrot cake.

❖ Cashews

In general, nuts are good sources of both protein and fiber, but they tend to be high in oil and fat. Cashews, how-

ever, are lower in fat than most other nuts. Over 50 percent
of their fat content is from unsaturated fatty acids, and 90
percent of that is from oleic acid, a monounsaturated oil.
Cashews have no cholesterol, but they do have 13 grams of
fat to the ounce. They also have a good amount of magnesium, potassium, zinc, and iron. Dry-roasted cashews have
about 163 calories to the ounce. (Cashews are always sold
shelled; the shells contain a caustic oil.)

Cook's Note

Avoid using cashews in cooked or baked dishes, as they
tend to become soggy. Cashews keep well, due to their high
oleic acid content. Store them in an airtight container in the
refrigerator for up to six months, or in the freezer for up to a
year.

See also Nuts.

❖ Cauliflower

One of the cruciferous (cabbagelike) vegetables, cauliflower has some potent health-giving nutrients. Along with
its cousins, broccoli and brussels sprouts, cauliflower contains sulfuraphane, a compound that can stimulate certain
enzymes that fight cancer within the body. Cauliflower may
be particularly useful for protecting you against breast and
colon cancer. This vegetable is also a very good source of
vitamin C and contains potassium, phosphorus, boron, and
lots of fiber, all for about 30 calories per cup. It's also a good
way to get your B vitamins, especially folic acid.

Cook's Note

Choose firm, white heads with no brown spots; pass up
any cauliflowers that are wilted or have a strong, cabbagelike odor. For a colorful addition to the dinner plate, try the

new green varieties (sometimes called broccoflowers). For the maximum beneficial effect, eat cauliflower raw or only lightly cooked.

❖ Celery

In many cultures, celery is a traditional remedy for high blood pressure. Until recently, modern doctors recommended against it, however, citing the high sodium level. Today, studies show that celery, despite its sodium content, contains a chemical that reduces the blood pressure in laboratory animals. (It also lowered the animals' cholesterol levels.) Two to four ribs of celery would be the human equivalent to the dosage a laboratory animal received. Celery has a lot of sodium for a vegetable, but the amount it contains as compared to other foods is still quite low—only about 35 milligrams a stalk. Celery is a good source of fiber, vitamin A, and potassium. There are only about 20 calories in a single stalk.

Celery is a mild diuretic that can be helpful for relieving mild water retention and breast tenderness of premenstrual stress (PMS). Celery also contains psoralens, compounds that may help relieve psoriasis symptoms.

Cook's Note

One medium celery stalk, chopped, yields about a cup. Select tight, pale-green heads with fresh-looking leaves. (The greener the celery, the more intense the flavor.) Steer clear of celery with limp stalks that bend. Always scrub the stalks before using. Celery can be stored for up to two weeks in the crisper section of the refrigerator. Wrap it in damp paper toweling and place it in a plastic bag to maintain optimum freshness.

❖ Cherries

There are two types of cherries: sweet (popular varieties include bing, black, Windsor, and Napoleon, to name a few), and sour (known as tart, pie, or red cherries). These stone fruits have their peak availability from May through August, although chewy dried cherries are now available year round. Fresh sweet cherries have only 5 calories each (or about 140 calories a cup), which makes them a satisfying treat for dieters. On average, water-soluble dietary fiber contributes 2.29 percent of the total weight of cherries. They're also a good source of vitamin A and potassium. Better still, recent research shows that cherries contain a substance known as ellagic acid, an antioxidant compound that helps keep your cells from becoming cancerous. Eating cherries also seems to help lower uric acid levels (useful if you have gout), and are quite effective in their ability to help prevent collagen destruction.

Cook's Note

Select plump, firm, glossy cherries with no bruises. Attached stems are a plus. To store, place cherries in a plastic bag (unwashed) and keep them in the refrigerator for up to four days.

❖ Chickpeas
(Garbanzo Beans or Ceci)

Round and yellow gold, chickpeas have a firm texture and slightly nutty flavor. They are one of the most nutritious members of the bean family, containing substantial amounts of protein, calcium, iron, and B vitamins. Chickpeas are a mainstay in Middle Eastern, Indian, and Mediterranean cooking.

Cook's Note

Dried chickpeas are very hard and require long soaking and long cooking. Try using canned chickpeas instead. Chickpeas are the main ingredient in popular Middle Eastern dishes such as hummus and falafel.

See also Beans.

❖ Chlorella

Chlorella is a food supplement made from a freshwater, unicellular green alga that contains an abundant amount of chlorophyll. A rich natural source of vitamin A, chlorophyll may help boost your immune system and help you resist infection. Chlorella also provides B vitamins, vitamin C, vitamin E, and minerals such as copper, iron, calcium, magnesium, and germanium. Chlorella tablets are sold in health food stores.

❖ Coconut

Despite its name, the coconut is not a nut at all. This fruit of the coconut palm tree is used extensively in Caribbean and Southeast Asian cuisines. It consists of over 50 percent water, 35 percent coconut oil, 10 percent carbohydrates, and a small amount of protein. Coconut is very high in fiber: 1

cup contains over 5 grams. But dieters beware: A cup of coconut meat has over 500 calories. Coconut oil is high in saturated fat and is often used in commercial baked goods (although it's not sold in the United States for home baking). The oil is also used in lotions, soaps, and shampoos.

Cook's Note

Choose coconuts that slosh when you shake them—that's the sound of coconut milk inside. To remove the coconut meat, first drain the nut of its liquid by piercing the "eyes" with a skewer or ice pick. Bake the coconut for 15 minutes at about 400 degrees F. This will shrink the meat from the shell for easier handling. Use a hammer to break open the coconut and remove the meat with a strong knife. (The brown membrane can be peeled off with a paring knife.) Use a grater or food processor to shred the meat. Commercial shredded coconut is often sweetened with sugar and preserved with propylene glycol (a colorless liquid used as a lubricant and as antifreeze). Coconut meat can be frozen for up to six months. A whole, uncracked coconut will keep at room temperature for about a month.

❖ Coffee

A passion for some people, an addiction for others, coffee has spawned quite a bit of controversy over the last few years. The controversy revolves around the caffeine found in coffee and its effect on the human body. At various times caffeine has been linked to heart disease, bladder cancer, breast cancer, birth defects, and other diseases. Generally, the proposed link is announced to much media fanfare, but when the studies later prove inconclusive, little attention is paid. In fact, there is no evidence that drinking coffee causes heart disease, cancer, high blood pressure, osteoporosis, high cholesterol, or any other serious ailment.

Caffeine is part of a group of naturally occurring compounds called methylxanthines. They're found in coffee beans, cola nuts, tea leaves, cocoa beans, and maté, a South American herbal drink. Caffeine stimulates the central nervous system. It is absorbed into the bloodstream within a few minutes and excreted in the urine after about three hours. Caffeine can cause insomnia for some people even in small amounts. In large amounts, it can cause nervousness, headaches, anxiety, irritability, and a slight rise in blood pressure. The effects of caffeine vary from individual to individual, however.

In general, caffeine is a safe and effective mild stimulant. A cup or two makes most people feel more alert and awake; a quiet cup of coffee or tea often helps relieve mild tension headaches. If caffeine keeps you from sleeping, avoid coffee, tea, and other caffeine-containing beverages for at least three hours before bedtime. If you have high blood pressure or heart disease (particularly any problems with irregular heartbeats), it is probably safe for you to take it in moderation (two cups a day), but you should discuss this with your doctor. Pregnant women are usually advised to avoid caffeine altogether, but recent studies suggest that moderate amounts of caffeine are not a problem. If you have gallstones or ulcers, it might be wise to avoid coffee—it could bring on an attack.

Caffeine is found in coffee (a 5-ounce brewed cup contains 115 milligrams; a 5-ounce percolated cup yields 80 milligrams); tea (40 to 60 milligrams per 5-ounce cup); carbonated soft drinks such as colas (30 to 45 milligrams per 12-ounce can), baking chocolate (26 milligrams in 1 ounce), and chocolate milk (5 milligrams in 8 ounces).

Decaffeinated coffee is specially processed to remove about 97 percent of the caffeine. Caffeine may be extracted by minimal amounts of methylene chloride (a controversial substance which has been found to cause cancer when inhaled in large amounts by lab animals) or by ethyl acetate (a naturally occurring substance in fruits and vegetables). Caffeine may also be removed by the Swiss water process. The coffee beans are steamed in water and the caffeine-containing outer layer is removed.

Cook's Note

Coffee flavor is determined by the type of bean used, the growing conditions (soil and climate), and how the bean was roasted. The darker the roast, the stronger the flavor. Store coffee beans in a cool, dark place; if you freeze them, do not defrost before using. Unopened containers of coffee last at least six months; once opened, they should be used within a month's time. A pound of coffee beans makes about forty cups of brewed coffee.

❖ Collard Greens

Rich in vitamin A and calcium, collard greens have large, silvery green, smooth leaves and tough stems. This leafy, green vegetable is a member of the cabbage family and is available fresh or frozen. A cup of raw, fresh collard greens has only 35 calories and just a trace of fat. They're a good source of calcium—1 cooked cup has 304 milligrams—and an excellent source of vitamin A—1 cooked cup has nearly 11,000 IU.

Cook's Note

Before cooking collard greens, chop off the tough stems and remove the center veins. Allow about 1/2 pound of uncooked greens per serving. Traditionally, collard greens were cooked Southern style: slowly, in a broth flavored with salt pork or ham. For a quicker and more healthful version, steam them briefly and then sauté lightly in olive oil, adding a touch of lemon juice or vinegar to enhance the flavor.

❖ Corn

A grain that provides complex carbohydrates, essential fatty acids, potassium, magnesium, vitamin A, vitamin C, and vitamin E, corn is also a great source of fiber. An ear of corn (about 1/2 cup of corn kernels) has just 77 calories, with 17 grams of carbohydrates, 2.4 grams of dietary fiber, and only a single gram of fat. Corn contains the B vitamins niacin, thiamine, and riboflavin, but it lacks two essential amino acids: lysine and tryptophan. Even so, it is a very nutritious food that is particularly valuable for vegetarians.

About half the world's corn crop is grown in the United States—some eight billion bushels a year. About 45 percent of that goes to animal feed, so every time you consume meat, eggs, dairy products, or milk, you're indirectly eating corn. Almost 6 percent of the American corn crop goes to make sweeteners. Only about 1.6 percent ends up on the table in the form of kernels, popcorn, or cornmeal, but that's still enough to be about four bushels a person every year.

Because corn has very little gluten, it's a good choice if you have celiac disease or wheat allergies. If you have irritable bowel syndrome, however, you might want to avoid corn. It often aggravates this condition.

Cook's Note

Fresh corn is at its peak availability from July to September. Canned and frozen kernels are readily available and very inexpensive. In addition to kernels, popular corn preparations include:

Cornmeal. Dried corn ground into a coarse flour. If possible, select stone-ground cornmeal. It retains more of the germ and oil and has a richer flavor. Cornmeal is used to make polenta, the Italian version of cornmeal mush.

Hominy. Large, whole corn kernels whose tough outer skins have been removed, usually by soaking the kernels in lye and water. Available canned and frozen.

Grits. Coarsely ground dried hominy, grits are a popular breakfast cereal.

Popcorn. Small, hard corn kernels that explode when heated. Leave off the butter for a low-calorie, high-fiber snack.

❖ Cranberries

Thanksgiving and Christmas meals seem to be the two occasions when cranberries are certain to make an appearance on the dining table, usually as some sort of relish. Aside from being festive, cranberries also have some medicinal value. Juice from these small, tart, reddish fruits is effective for treating and preventing urinary tract infections. For years, doctors thought it worked because the acidity of cranberry juice made the urine more acidic. Recent studies show, however, that cranberry juice inhibits the growth of harmful bacteria by keeping them from adhering to the lining of the bladder and urethra. If you think you have a urinary tract infection, see your doctor. Antibiotics will usually clear it up in just a day or so. If you get urinary tract infections often, having a daily glass of cranberry juice may reduce their frequency and severity.

Cook's Note
Fresh, unsweetened cranberry juice is usually only available at health food stores. The commercially prepared cranberry juice sold in supermarkets is heavily sweetened with corn syrup and diluted somewhat with water, although it will still help urinary tract infections. If the natural, unsweetened version is too tart for you, mix it with apple, pear, or grape juices. Cranberries are sold fresh from October through December. Unopened packages can be stored in the freezer for up to twelve months for year-round use.

❖ Cucumber

A vine vegetable native to India, cucumbers are delicious as munching snacks, crudités, or in salads. The dark green skin contains most of the cucumber's nutrients: traces of vitamins and minerals, along with silica, a mineral necessary for strong connective tissues. Cucumbers also contain sterols, compounds that could help lower your blood cholesterol level. The pulp of a cucumber is mostly water. To reduce puffiness and revive tired eyes, try placing cool cucumber slices on your eyes. A typical seven-inch cucumber has fewer than 30 calories.

Cook's Note
Supermarket cucumbers are usually waxed to slow spoilage and should be peeled before eating. But since all of the nutrients are in the skin, try buying unwaxed, organic cucumbers at the health food store instead. Kirby cucumbers, used for pickling, are never waxed. European or seedless English cucumbers are generally sold wrapped in plastic instead of being waxed, but they are usually more expensive than regular cucumbers. Choose dark green, firm cucumbers; they will keep for up to two weeks in the refrigerator. A large cucumber may have lots of tough seeds. To remove them, slice the cucumber lengthwise and then scrape away the seeds with a spoon.

❖ Dandelion

The bane of gardeners, dandelion is treasured by natural healers and herbalists. This weed is rich in nutrients that could help improve liver and gallbladder function. The greens are rich in beta carotene and vitamin C, two antioxidants that can help protect against heart disease and cancer, and contain goodly amounts of B vitamins, calcium, iron, magnesium, and zinc as well. Dandelion greens act as a mild diuretic, while the root has a slight laxative effect.

Cook's Note

Fresh dandelion greens are usually available in spring, in green markets, health food stores, and supermarkets. They have a pleasant, bittersweet taste. Choose small, tender leaves and combine them in salads with other, milder greens such as iceberg lettuce or Belgian endive. Juice the entire dandelion with other vegetables, such as carrots, for a refreshing and healthy drink.

❖ Dates

High in calories (1 cup of this rich, sweet fruit contains about 500 calories) and high in complex carbohydrates, dates have no fat or sodium. They are an excellent source of dietary fiber: a cup of dried dates has over 4 grams. This energy-rich food also contains calcium, iron, potassium, and phosphorus, along with several important B vitamins. Dates have been an important food source throughout human history. In fact, the date palm is considered to be the first cultivated tree. Research suggests that date palms grew along the Nile as early as the fifth century B.C. Dates are still a staple food in the Middle East and North Africa.

Cook's Note

There are several varieties of dates. Whichever you choose, dates should always be plump and glossy. In the

United States, most dates come from California. The most popular varieties are:

Deglet Noor (date of light). Semisoft and amber-colored, this is the date most commonly sold.

Zahidi (nobility). These dates are smaller, more golden-toned, and more egg-shaped than Deglet Noor.

Khadrawy (green). These soft dates are harvested by hand.

Halawy (sweet). Also soft, these dates have a slightly sweeter taste than Khadrawy dates.

❖ Eggplant

A member of the nightshade family, eggplant gets its name from the white variety, which resembles an egg in shape. Low in calories and virtually fat-free, eggplant is a fabulous source of minerals. For only 25 calories per 1/2 cup, you get calcium, potassium, magnesium, and iron, with just a trace of sodium. There are reports that eggplant helps lower cholesterol levels and is a digestive aid. It is also being investigated by the National Cancer Institute for its potential anticancer properties, particularly against a form of skin cancer called basal cell carcinoma.

Cook's Note

Eggplant rapidly absorbs the flavors of the herbs and spices it is cooked with; unfortunately, it is also a sponge for any kind of oil or butter. "Oven-frying" eggplant in a small amount of oil is a good way to cut back on the amount of oil it absorbs. If you must sauté it, salt the eggplant beforehand and it will soak up less oil. Look for firm eggplants with glossy, bruise-free skin. Eggplant stays fresh, refrigerated, for up to five days; less-than-fresh eggplant has a bitter flavor. European and Asian eggplants have an edible purple skin and creamy interior pulp; the white-skinned variety has a sweeter interior but should always be eaten peeled. All eggplant should be cooked before eating.

❖ Eggs

Many health-conscious people have become almost phobic about eating eggs, thinking that they are crammed with dangerous fat and cholesterol. In fact, one large egg does contain 213 milligrams of cholesterol and 5 grams of fat, all of which is found in the yolk. Yet eating foods that contain cholesterol probably won't raise your blood cholesterol. Generally, your body will simply produce less to keep your level about the same. To be on the safe side, however, follow the American Heart Association's recommendation: up to four whole eggs (or egg yolks) per week for people on cholesterol-lowering diets. And since the whites are both fat-free and cholesterol-free, they can be eaten without limit.

Liquid egg substitutes are all based on egg whites, and each brand uses a different formula to replace the yolks. Read the labels for nutrient information.

Cook's Note

It is possible to get salmonella (food poisoning) from eggs that have been improperly handled. Salmonella can cause serious illness or even death, especially in children, the elderly, and people with impaired immune systems. To avoid salmonella from eggs, keep them refrigerated and cook them thoroughly. Buy AA or A graded eggs from the refrigerator case, get them home quickly, and refrigerate them immediately. Keep them refrigerated until you're ready to use them. Discard any eggs that are unclean, cracked, broken, or leaking. Do not eat products made with raw eggs (hollandaise sauce, mayonnaise, eggnogs, home-made ice cream, Caesar salads, or any raw batters).

Eggs are a staple in most kitchens, valued for their role in leavening baked goods and binding together ingredients. For safety's sake, remember that salmonella organisms will not survive if held at 140 degrees F. for 3 1/2 minutes, or if the food reaches an end-point temperature of 160 degrees F. For soft-cooked eggs, follow the American Egg Board's recommendation: Bring the eggs and water to a boil, then turn off the heat. Cover the pot and let stand about four or five minutes. Make sure your hands, utensils, and work surfaces are clean. Avoid mixing yolks and whites with the shells when breaking or separating eggs—use an inexpensive egg separator instead.

❖ Fava Beans (Broad Beans)

A type of shell bean, fava beans are large, flat beans shaped a little like lima beans. They range in color from white to brown. These beans are a staple food in Egypt and the Middle East, and are popular in Italian cooking as well. In the spring, you'll sometimes see fresh fava beans in their pods at the supermarket or green market, but usually fava beans are sold in dried form. Like other beans, fava beans are high in protein and fiber and low in fat. There are only 93 calories per 1/2 cup of cooked dried beans; that same 1/2 cup provides 5 grams of fiber—about one-quarter of the recommended daily intake.

A fairly rare condition called favism can cause red blood cells to rupture after you eat fava beans or inhale the pollen. This genetic defect affects up to 35 percent of some Mediterranean populations and about 10 percent of African-

Americans. Favism symptoms can include fatigue, nausea, vomiting, dizziness, and severe anemia.

Cook's Note

Fava beans need a long soaking and take about one hour to cook.

❖ Fennel (Finocchio)

With its feathery cap of leaves and celerylike stalks, fennel looks a lot like dill, but it tastes a lot like anise or licorice. Its stems are low in calories (only 56 in 1/2 pound) and high in vitamin A (1/2 pound has 7,000 IU) and potassium (about 750 milligrams). Fennel is also a good source of dietary fiber.

Chewing on fennel seeds can freshen your breath. Tea made from fennel seeds is traditionally recommended for promoting milk in breast-feeding mothers (although it is probably the additional liquid, not the fennel itself, that helps). Fennel seed tea can help settle an upset stomach and relieve indigestion. A few drops added to the bottle can often calm a colicky baby.

Cook's Note

Fennel is fairly easy to find in green markets and large supermarkets. Choose crisp, white bulbs and stalks, avoiding any that have soft areas or brown bruises. Store fennel in a plastic bag in the refrigerator for up to two days. It's delicious raw as crudités, and it's often braised until just tender and served as a side dish. Try adding some fennel seeds to marinades for chicken and seafood.

❖ Figs

Sometimes sold fresh but mostly sold dried, figs can make a valuable contribution to a healthful diet. Dried figs have the highest dietary fiber content of any common fruit, nut, or vegetable. Consequently, they are very effective for relieving constipation. They provide a good source of calcium (there's 53 milligrams in a 1.4-ounce serving), and potassium (244 milligrams in a serving), as well as magnesium and iron. Figs have about 20 to 40 calories each (depending on the variety) and are lower in calories per gram of dietary fiber than other fruits. They also are higher in pectin, a type of dietary fiber, than many other fruits. Figs are traditionally recommended as an aid to digestion. The natural sugars in figs (dextrose and fructose) pump quick energy into the blood—great for an energy-boosting snack. If you're subject to migraines, however, eat figs sparingly or avoid them altogether. They are a headache trigger for some people.

Cook's Note

Delicate fresh figs are harvested when ripe, then rushed to stores, where they should be consumed within eight days or so. Refrigerate and use as soon as possible. Dried figs make an intriguing, zesty salad when combined with walnuts and mixed greens. The two most common varieties of dried figs are amber-colored Calimyrna and dark-fleshed Black Mission.

❖ Fish and Fish Oil

Because fish is low in fat and calories and high in protein, doctors and nutritionists have long recommended it. A 3-ounce serving of any lean, white-fleshed fish, such as flounder, sole, red snapper, or sea bass, contains just a single gram of fat and fewer than 100 calories. Fattier, oily fish, such as tuna, catfish, salmon, bluefish, and trout, are slightly higher in calories and contain anywhere from 3 to 7 grams of fat per serving. Substituting a serving of fish for a serving of lean T-bone steak, for example, would save some 100 calories and 8 grams of fat. In fact, over 70 percent of the calories in a serving of lean T-bone steak come from fat, while only about half the calories in a serving of sea bass come from fat.

But eating fish has benefits beyond cutting calories and fat. Omega-3 fatty acid, or fish oil, is used by your body to make eicosapentanoic acid (EPA), which in turn is needed to make prostaglandins, hormonelike substances that, among other things, help discourage heart disease by keeping your blood flowing normally, preventing the buildup of plaque in your arteries, and reducing the chances of dangerous blood clots. Fish oil can also raise your HDL (good) cholesterol and lower your triglyceride levels, and it can help lower your blood pressure.

Fish oil is a polyunsaturated fat, found in all seafood (but especially deep-sea fatty fish); fatty fishes also contain pre-formed EPA. According to the National Heart and Lung Institute, a single gram of omega-3 fatty acids daily (about the amount in a 3-ounce serving of fish) could reduce the risk of cardiovascular disease in men. Just how substantial the reduction might be is somewhat controversial. A recent study of American men who routinely ate fish two or three times a week showed no reduction in their rate of cardiovascular disease, even when other factors, such as cigarette smoking and exercise, were taken into account. While there's no guarantee that eating more fish will keep you from having a heart attack, it is possible that eating more fish could improve your overall health by helping you eat less saturated fat. Fish can also be a source of valuable nutrients. Canned salmon and sardines (with the bones) are a good way to add calcium to your diet.

Supplemental fish oil capsules, found in health food stores, are rather expensive and don't offer much in the way of culinary satisfaction. A fresh piece of fish that has been poached, steamed, or lightly sautéed is a much more delicious way to reap the same benefits. Below is a list of some fish favorites.

Anchovy. A 3 1/2-ounce serving has 127 calories and 4.8 grams of fat, including 1.4 grams of omega-3 fatty acid. These little fish are also rich in nucleic acids, which some researchers believe may help retard the aging process.

Cod. A 4-ounce serving has only 118 calories and 37 milligrams of cholesterol.

Flounder and sole. There are only 80 calories in a 3-ounce serving, with just one gram of fat. Flounder and sole are almost impossible to tell apart: they are both mild-tasting flat fish.

Mackerel. One of the most potent sources of omega-3 fatty acids—a 4-ounce serving has a whopping 2.1 grams. Mackerel is also high in calcium; vitamins A, D, and E; niacin; B_{12}; and riboflavin.

Orange roughy. This mild, firm-fleshed white fish is usually sold frozen in steaks or fillets. Orange roughy is virtually fat-free; a 4-ounce serving has just 100 calories.

Red snapper. Low in calories and fat, a 3-ounce serving has just 100 calories, with 1.3 grams of fat and 37 milligrams of cholesterol.

Salmon. The full-flavored, firm, pink flesh of salmon is available in several varieties. Coho or Atlantic is usually sold fresh, while red or sockeye is usually found in cans. Atlantic salmon contains 2.1 grams of omega-3 fatty acid in a 4-ounce serving. Canned salmon (with bone) is a rich source of calcium and vitamin D. All varieties are low in calories and cholesterol.

Sardines. Canned in oil, sardines provide 0.7 grams of omega-3 fatty acid and 10 percent of the RDA for calcium in a 4-ounce serving. They also contain nucleic acids (RNA and DNA), which some researchers believe may retard the aging process.

Sea bass. Low in saturated fat and calories, sea bass has a half gram of omega-3 fatty acid in a 4-ounce serving.

Shrimp. Though not a fish (technically speaking, they're related to spiders), shrimp is a healthful and very popular seafood. One 3-ounce serving of shrimp has 450 milligrams of omega-3 fatty acid.

Tuna. Perhaps the most popular fish, tuna is a rich source of omega-3 fatty acid—about 1.2 grams in a 3-ounce serving of fresh bluefin tuna. Canned light tuna in water, however, has only about 100 milligrams in a serving. Tuna is also a good source of selenium and vitamin D.

❖ Garlic

A member of the lily family and related to the onion, garlic has been used in cooking for over 5,000 years. Over the centuries, it has also acquired a reputation in folk medicine as a laxative, diuretic, sedative, and antiseptic, and been touted as a remedy for a multitude of maladies, including gastrointestinal disorders, animal bites, hemorrhoids, ulcers, loss of appetite, tumors, and heart disease. It's even been considered an aphrodisiac. The truth is almost as remarkable: garlic contains numerous compounds that have been shown to help prevent heart disease, stroke, cancer, high cholesterol, and infections. To get the maximum protective effects of garlic, doctors recommend two or three cloves a day, raw or cooked.

Garlic as an Antibiotic

In both world wars, doctors were forced to improvise when medical supplies ran short. They discovered that garlic is a potent antibiotic, and it helped heal wounds. In Russia, garlic is known as Russian penicillin, and 500 tons were once rushed there to deal with an influenza outbreak. Allicin, the odoriferous compound that releases its pungent odor when garlic is cut or crushed, was once thought to be the source of garlic's benefits. In fact, it is the sulfur-containing compounds formed by the breakdown of allicin that have the pharmacological effects.

Garlic as a Heart Helper

By reducing your blood's clotting ability (lessening the stickiness of blood platelets), garlic helps prevent the formation of life-threatening blood clots. Garlic can also help improve blood cholesterol levels by lowering your LDL (bad) cholesterol level and raising your HDL (good) cholesterol level. It can also help lower your level of the potentially harmful blood fats known as triglycerides.

Garlic as an Anticancer Aid

Animal studies suggest that garlic can help protect you against cancer caused by exposure to carcinogens. Other studies indicate that garlic may help prevent metastasis, or the spread of cancer cells from their original site to other parts of your body. Garlic contains some fifteen potent antioxidant substances that help protect you from cancer and other diseases.

Garlic as a Blood Pressure Stabilizer

The Japanese government officially recognizes garlic as a blood-pressure depressor. In laboratory animals, garlic consistently lowers blood pressure levels. Studies on humans have also shown a drop in systolic and diastolic blood pressure when garlic was consumed.

Garlic as a Common Cold Fighter

Garlic seems to work the way most over-the-counter expectorants and decongestants do: it irritates the stomach, signaling the lungs to release fluids that thin out mucus, which helps your lungs expel it.

Cook's Note

Buy firm, fresh garlic bulbs (heads) and store them in a cool, dry, dark place. Avoid bulbs that are soft or are beginning to sprout. Remove cloves as needed. Since eating garlic (especially raw garlic) can be hazardous to your breath, try chewing some fresh parsley sprigs or a few fennel seeds. Garlic supplements, such as Kyolic, are sold as liquids or as odorless capsules containing dried garlic. If you don't like the taste of garlic, try taking the supplements instead.

❖ Grapefruit

Low in calories, fat, and sodium, grapefruit is a natural source of many nutrients. The membrane between grapefruit segments contains pectin, a form of soluble fiber that has been shown to help lower blood cholesterol levels. Like other citrus fruits, grapefruit contains flavonoids, substances that are antioxidants and may help prevent cancer and heart disease. It also contains substances called lycopene and limonene, which have significantly reduced tumors in laboratory animals. Grapefruit is a rich source of vitamin C, which may bolster your immune system and help ward off colds. A grapefruit half has only 40 calories. Despite claims, grapefruit can't magically burn off fat. In fact, the so-called grapefruit diet can actually be harmful. Discuss any weight-loss diet with your doctor before you try it.

Cook's Note

Once available only in winter, grapefruit is now available year round. Here are several of the most popular varieties:

White or Golden. This is the traditional grapefruit. It has bright yellow skin with firm, slightly tart fruit.

Ruby Red. Otherwise known as pink grapefruit, this variety has yellow skin with a red blush. The fruit is pink and sweet.

Pummelo (also called Chinese grapefruit). A very large grapefruit with thick yellow skin. White or pink inside, it is less acidic than other grapefruits.

Melogold and *Oro Blanco.* Both are crosses between a grapefruit and a Pummelo, and both have fruit that is sweeter than regular white grapefruit.

Ruby Star and *Rio Red.* Yellow red on the outside, both varieties have a deep red blush on the skin and a deeper-colored interior fruit than Ruby Red.

❖ Grapes

The world's leading food crop and one of the oldest cultivated crops (since 5000 B.C.), grapes provide some remarkable health benefits. Originally it was believed that red wine helped thin the blood by discouraging blood platelets from clumping together, thereby reducing blood clots that can lead to heart attacks or strokes. But now researchers believe that it's a compound in the skins of red (but not white) grapes, resveratrol, that provides the benefit. Grapes provide other health benefits as well. Grapes contain boron, a mineral your body needs to help retain calcium. Getting enough boron can help slow or prevent the bone loss of osteoporosis. Grapes also contain ellagic acid, which has been shown to combat cancer; they're also a good source of vitamin C and some of the B vitamins. A cup of green Thompson seedless grapes has 114 calories (or about 3 calories per grape), with only a trace of fat and sodium. The same cup provides 1.1 grams of dietary fiber.

Cook's Note

Today, grapes are available year round. Look for firm, vibrantly colored grapes that are still attached to their stems. Store them unwashed in loose paper towels in the refrigerator. Rinse grapes before eating. For an enjoyable hot-weather treat, try eating frozen grapes. A number of grape varieties are offered.

Thompson seedless. These are the popular pale-green, seedless grapes most frequently seen in supermarkets. The more yellow green they are, the sweeter they taste.

Red Flame seedless. This is a popular red variety—the redder the better.

Emperor. These red grapes are smaller and sometimes darker in color than Red Flame. They are seedless and very thin-skinned.

Concord. Often grown in backyard arbors, these grapes have a deep blue-black color, seeds, and tough skins. Although they are very good eaten as is, they tend to be tart and are usually made into jams or jellies.

Ribier. These grapes are also blue black, but are usually larger than Concord. They have a sweet, mild flavor.

Champagne. Tiny, delicious, and sweet, these grapes are a bit of a rarity. You can eat them as is or use them as a beautiful garnish for a festive platter (and eat them later).

❖ Guava

A sweet tropical fruit, one guava has nearly three times the recommended dietary allowance for vitamin C (165 milligrams). A single guava has about 46 calories and a hefty 4.9 grams of dietary fiber. Guava also contains a good amount of potassium (255 milligrams) and beta carotene.

Cook's Note

Select smooth, bruise-free guavas (the skin can vary in color from pale yellow to yellow green) that have a rich aroma. If the guava is ripe, the skin will yield to gentle pressure. Canned guava juice is not a particularly good substitute for the fresh fruit—it frequently has added sweeteners and may contain artificial coloring.

❖ Hazelnuts (Filberts)

Hazelnuts, with their sweet, rich flavor, are often added to baked goods. They're also used to flavor liqueurs such as Frangelico. But in terms of health, the chief virtue of hazelnuts is their fat content—the good kind. No other food has a higher percentage of monounsaturated fat, which can help protect you against heart disease. Of the fat in a hazelnut, 81 percent is monounsaturated; by comparison, only 72 percent of the fat in olive oil is. Hazelnuts are also a good dietary source of boron.

❖ Honey

A natural sweetener, honey is made by honeybees from flower nectar. The flavor and color of honey depends on the flowers used to produce it. Many people feel that because honey is a natural, unrefined product, it is somehow better for you than refined table sugar, but this is not so. In fact, a tablespoon of honey contains about 64 calories, roughly 20 more calories than an equivalent amount of white table sugar. Honey is made mostly of sucrose, exactly the same substance as table sugar (although honey also contains fructose and glucose). If you should avoid sweeteners such as sugar (if you have diabetes, for example), you should also avoid honey.

Because honey contains antimicrobial substances, it has been used for centuries to treat minor wounds and burns. While the honey may temporarily soothe the sore skin, it's not really beneficial—you're better off just keeping the area clean with soap and water. (Never try to treat severe or infected wounds and burns with honey. See your doctor instead.) A traditional remedy for coughs and sore throats is a syrup made of honey and garlic.

Honey contains no fat or sodium and only insignificant amounts of minerals.

Never give honey to infants under one year. Honey is an unsterilized product and can foster the growth of botulism, which can cause death in babies. Older children and adults are not usually affected.

Cook's Note

Store honey at room temperature in a tightly covered container. Refrigerating honey can cause crystallization. To liquefy crystallized honey, place the jar in a pan of warm (not hot) water until the honey liquefies.

❖ Horseradish

A pungent root vegetable related to mustard, horseradish is available fresh in the produce section of supermarkets from fall through spring. Originally from eastern Europe and western Asia, horseradish was once thought to help alleviate asthma. Today, it is used to give dishes a fiery flavor and as an appetite stimulant. Horseradish is also valuable as a decongestant for relieving cold, flu, and sinusitis symptoms. An old folk remedy for stuffy noses, sore throats, and coughs is a hot mixture of honey, grated horseradish, and hot water.

Cook's Note

Fresh horseradish root can be stored in a plastic bag in the refrigerator for up to two weeks. Commercially prepared horseradish can be found in the refrigerated dairy section. White horseradish is prepared with vinegar, the milder red variety contains beet juice. Prepared horseradish will keep in the refrigerator for up to four months, but it will lose some of its potency in that time. Grate fresh horseradish just before using for best flavor.

❖ Hot Peppers (Chili Peppers or Cayenne Pepper)

Hot peppers are an authentic American food. Although they were unknown to the rest of the world before Columbus, today, fiery hot peppers are an integral part of many ethnic cuisines and have acquired a growing legion of fans. Prized for their spicy heat, these peppers are not only good, they're good for you.

Technically speaking, hot peppers are berries, the fruit of shrubs in the *Capsicum* genus. A single hot pepper contains a full day's supply of beta carotene and nearly twice the recommended dietary allowance for vitamin C. (Bell peppers and paprika, sweet members of the *Capsicum* genus, also have large amounts of these vitamins.)

Hot peppers get their bite from a compound called capsaicin. When applied to the skin, capsaicin can block pain impulses. For this reason, ointments containing capsaicin are used to relieve the pain of shingles; they have also been used to some effect for treating psoriasis and arthritis. Capsaicin is also the substance behind some other valuable uses for hot peppers. It can help lower your LDL (bad) blood cholesterol and reduce your triglyceride levels. Hot peppers may also keep your blood from forming dangerous clots that could lead to a heart attack or stroke. Hot peppers help stimulate gastric juices, so they are an effective appetite stimulant as well as making food more flavorful. The capsaicin in hot peppers can also help clear up stuffy noses and congested bronchial tubes. Despite what people say, hot peppers do not cause ulcers or gallbladder problems.

Once found only in ethnic markets and gourmet shops, numerous hot pepper varieties are now available in any large supermarket. Some of the most popular are:

Anaheim. Long, narrow, and green, this is one of the mildest hot peppers.

Ancho. This dark brown, dried poblano chili with a slightly nutty flavor has a heat content that can range from mild to medium-hot.

Chipotle. Available canned or dried, chipotles are smoked and dried jalapeño peppers.

Jalapeño. This short, medium-hot green pepper is readily available fresh, canned, or pickled.

Poblano. This pepper is long and irregularly shaped with mild to medium-hot flavor.

Serrano. Tiny, thin, and red or green in color, they are very hot and are frequently used in salsa.

Cook's Note

Avoid touching your eyes, mouth, and nose when handling hot peppers; the oils can be very irritating. Wear thin plastic gloves or plastic bags over your hands, and always wash your hands thoroughly after handling hot peppers.

❖ Jerusalem Artichokes

The name of this tuber is misleading, for it isn't an artichoke at all. Related to the sunflower, the Jerusalem artichoke is a member of the daisy family. Native to North America, it is sometimes called sunchoke. The word *Jerusalem* in its name is actually a corruption of the Spanish word *girasol,* which means *turning toward the sun.* Jerusalem artichokes are rich sources of a starch called inulin. Although your body doesn't metabolize inulin, this substance helps promote the growth of beneficial bacteria in your intestinal tract. These bacteria help inhibit disease-causing organisms and may help lower serum cholesterol levels. Inulin may also provide some immune-enhancing benefits as well and can be helpful for controlling blood sugar levels in diabetics. Additionally, Jerusalem artichokes provide iron (one of the few vegetable sources that do), thiamine, potassium, and folate.

Cook's Note
Jerusalem artichoke tubers should be large and firm. They keep well in the refrigerator for up to two weeks. Peel them and eat them raw as crudités or in salads. They can also be baked or fried much like potatoes.

❖ Kale

Kale is a leafy member of the cabbage (cruciferous) family; it is closely related to collard greens. The difference is that kale features curly-edged leaves and is not as heat tolerant. With about 9,000 IU of beta carotene per cooked cup, kale contains more than spinach does. A single cup of it also provides enough vitamin C to exceed the RDA. That same cup has more calcium than an equivalent amount of milk, and your body can absorb it better. A good source of iron, magnesium, and potassium, kale is also a good way to get dietary fiber—1 cup provides about 3 grams. Powerful cancer-fighting compounds called indoles are also found in kale.

Cook's Note

Kale is blue-green, chewy, and has a mildly bitter but pleasant taste. All parts of the plant are edible, but most cooks cut away the tough stems. Kale keeps for up to one week refrigerated in a plastic bag.

❖ Kidney Beans (Habichuelas or Chili Beans)

Just 1/2 cup of cooked dark-red kidney beans provides about 100 calories and a whopping 7 grams of dietary fiber. Kidney beans have barely a trace of fat and only a tiny amount of sodium. One serving of kidney beans also supplies nearly half the recommended daily requirement for folic acid, about a quarter of the recommended daily allowance for iron, and a good dose of magnesium, potassium, thiamine, vitamin B_6, and zinc.

Cook's Note

Kidney beans are an essential ingredient in many bean dishes, including Southern-style red beans and rice and Southwestern chili.

See also Beans.

❖ Kiwifruit

Native to New Zealand, this small, oval, fuzzy brown fruit has a dazzlingly green interior that is sweet, juicy, and bursting with vitamin C and potassium. A single fruit has 46 calories, and about 2.6 grams of dietary fiber, with just a tiny amount of fat (less then 1/2 gram) and sodium (only 4 milligrams). The small black seeds are edible, but remove the brown skin.

Cook's Note

Kiwifruit (also known as kiwi) should be about as firm as a ripe pear. To ripen kiwifruit, leave it at room temperature until it is the right softness, then place it in your refrigerator; it will keep there for up to a week.

❖ Leeks

Closely related to onions and garlic (members of the *Allium* genus), leeks have a long, narrow bulb with long, green leaves and stem. The bulb is not eaten; the leaves and stem are. Like other members of the *Allium* genus, leeks contain compounds that may help protect you against stomach cancer, and they can also help lower your blood cholesterol level. At a mere 16 calories per 1/2 cup, leeks also provide 1.3 grams of dietary fiber.

Cook's Note

Leeks are even milder than scallions. Choose bright green, moist leaves; avoid any bulbs that look old or shriveled. Leeks keep in the refrigerator in a plastic bag for up to five days. The leaves and stalk can collect a lot of dirt, so clean the leek thoroughly by slicing it lengthwise and rinsing it under cold, running water. Be sure to expose all the leaves to the water. Use as you would onions, by slicing or chopping and adding to dishes to be cooked or baked.

❖ Lemon

A tart, bright yellow citrus fruit, grown mostly in California and Florida, lemons are available year round. The juice from half a lemon (about 2 tablespoons) provides a little more than 25 percent of the Recommended Dietary Allowance of vitamin C.

Cook's Note

Lemons keep in the refrigerator for up to three weeks. Look for glossy, fine-textured skins; avoid spongy textures or lemons with soft spots at the stem. A good lemon should feel heavy for its size. To get the most juice from a lemon, microwave it for about 10 seconds on high, or roll it on the counter with the palm of your hand.

❖ Lentils

One of the oldest cultivated plants on earth, lentils are rich in iron (you get 33 percent of the recommended daily allowance in a cooked 1/2 cup) and contain 25 percent protein. These tiny, round, flat legumes are also high in dietary fiber (about 5 grams in a cooked 1/2 cup) and they're also especially rich in folic acid—you get nearly 90 percent of the recommended daily allowance in a cooked 1/2 cup. Lentils also have healthy doses of iron, potassium, and copper, and phytates, compounds that may help prevent cancerous changes in cells.

Cook's Note

A staple in many ethnic cuisines, lentils need no soaking and cook up in just 15 to 20 minutes. (Watch them carefully—they can become mushy if overcooked.) Types of lentils include brown lentils, which are most often used in making soups; green lentils (also called Egyptian lentils), which are frequently served in salads; and red lentils, which are often sold as split lentils, and have an orange hue when cooked. They are chiefly used for soups, stews, and purees. Masoor dal is a staple of Indian and Middle Eastern cooking; this bean dish is made with lentils that have had their seed coats removed and thus cook very quickly.

See also Beans.

❖ Lettuce

There are many types of lettuce, but the rule of thumb is this: The darker the leaf, the better the lettuce is for you. Although lettuce is high in fiber, some of its best qualities are what it *doesn't* possess: fat, calories, or sodium. There are minor differences among the greens. Here's a breakdown:

Arugula. Also called rocket, roquette, or rogula, this snappy green has a distinctive peppery taste. An excellent source of vitamin A, vitamin C, and calcium.

Endive. Creamy white, oblong, and firm, with small, tight heads, endive (also called Belgian endive) has a mild flavor.

Romaine (cos lettuce). This leafy green is number one on the best greens list. It grows in dark green, oblong heads with a distinctive vertical rib. Romaine is a very good source of beta carotene: a single cup gives you nearly one-quarter of your recommended dietary allowance of vitamin C. Romaine is also a good source of folic acid and potassium—1 cup has 9 calories.

Leaf lettuce. The darker the leaves on this green, the higher the beta carotene content. It grows in loose, leafy heads; some varieties have a reddish tinge. One cup of leaf lettuce has 10 calories.

Butterhead or Boston. With only 5 calories per cup, butterhead lettuce has some folic acid and small amounts of beta carotene and vitamin C.

Iceberg. One of the most common salad greens, iceberg lettuce is fairly dense, so eating a cupful is actually somewhat filling. Iceberg has a healthy amount of folic acid as well as vitamin C, iron, and potassium.

Cook's Note

To get the full benefits of lettuce, avoid drowning it in high-fat, high-calorie salad dressings.

❖ Lima Beans (Butter Beans or Pole Beans)

Lima beans pack 23 percent protein, 6.8 grams of dietary fiber, and quite a bit of folic acid (39 percent of the recommended daily allowance) into each 1/2-cup serving. Lima beans contain virtually no fat or sodium; they have about 108 calories per 1/2-cup serving. They're also a good source of iron, potassium, calcium, phosphorus, magnesium, and B vitamins.

Cook's Note

Lima beans are somewhat flat and range in color from creamy white to pale green. There are two varieties: the large lima is about 1 1/4 inches long; the small lima (baby or sieva) is only about 1/2 inch long. There is no difference in taste or texture, but small limas have a somewhat thinner skin and so cook a bit more quickly. Bland and soft-textured, dried lima beans are often used to make a puree that is delicious with lamb.

❖ Lime

Similar in nutritional value to lemons, limes are a citrus fruit originally grown in Southeast Asia. Aside from their tart flavor, their chief benefit is a good amount of vitamin C.

Cook's Note

At their best, limes should have a smooth, shiny green skin with no bruises or brown spots. Limes are quite perishable; they last in the refrigerator for no longer than two weeks.

❖ Liver

Nutritionally speaking, there is good and bad news about liver. The good news is that it is extremely rich in vitamin A, vitamin B$_{12}$, and other B vitamins. Three ounces of cooked chicken or calf's liver also contains three times the Recommended Dietary Allowance of folic acid. Liver is also a very good source of iron and is often recommended for anemic people and women with very heavy menstrual periods. Finally, it contributes both zinc and vitamin C to your diet. The bad news is that 3 ounces of cooked liver contribute nearly double the recommended daily allowance for your total cholesterol consumption. In addition, since any medicines, hormones, or other additives that were fed to the animal tend to accumulate in the liver, you may also be eating these unwanted substances.

Cook's Note

Liver is highly perishable, so it's important to choose fresh liver and use it within twenty-four hours. Select bright, shiny liver and wipe it clean with a damp cloth before cooking. (Remove the thin outer layer of skin beforehand.) Cook liver gently. Don't overcook—it will get tough.

❖ Melons

Melons fall into two categories: muskmelons and winter melons. Muskmelons, of which cantaloupe is a prime example, have a raised, netted skin that is lighter in color than the skin underneath. These melons have a strong aroma and a short shelf life. Winter melons, including casaba, Persian, crenshaw, and honeydew, have smoother skins and no netting; their skin is sometimes striped. Winter melons have very little scent and will keep for longer than muskmelons. Watermelons are in a class of their own, with their bright red flesh, potentially enormous size, and their concentration of lycopenes, a cancer-fighting antioxidant.

All melons, especially those with golden flesh, are rich in vitamin A, and many are also a good to excellent source of vitamin C. In fact, one serving of cantaloupe (half a melon) offers 50 percent of the RDA for vitamin A and more than 100 percent of the RDA for vitamin C. Cantaloupe also provides potassium and folic acid. Women who are pregnant or trying to conceive are encouraged to eat yellow or orange fruits for their folic acid; cantaloupe definitely falls into this category.

Melons are also low in calories. Half a cantaloupe contains only 93 calories; a wedge of honeydew (about one-fifth of a melon) has only 45.

Below is a rundown of the most popular melon varieties:

Cantaloupe. This popular melon has netted skin over a green-gray to light yellowish rind. The stem end is slightly indented, round, and smooth, and the melon should have a refreshingly sweet aroma. The flesh is golden orange, juicy, and sweet.

Casaba. The hallmark of this melon is a rough, wrinkled rind that is golden over green when ripe. The melon is somewhat pointed at one end. The flesh is smooth and creamy white to pale green. Some say it tastes something like a mango.

Crenshaw. The rind on this melon has blotches of yellow green or gold when ripe. A cross between a casaba and a cantaloupe, the flesh is very juicy, sweet, and tender; it is golden to light pink in color.

Honeydew. The smooth, hard rind is the color of heavy cream with pale-yellow undertones. The stem end has a smooth indentation and the blossom end emits a musky scent. This melon is aptly named: the pale green flesh is extremely sweet. Orange-fleshed varieties are available.

Persian. Netted skin over a green to gray rind that darkens as it ripens characterize this melon. The blossom end should be just soft and smell sweet. The pink orange flesh has a slightly spicy undertone.

Cook's Note

Melons do not ripen after being picked, so check the stem end carefully before you buy. If the melon was picked before being fully ripe, the scar at the stem end will be well callused. Select melons that are heavy for their size and sound solid when lightly tapped.

See also Watermelon.

❖ Milk

Milk is one of the oldest health foods, famed for its many nutritional benefits, which is why "Drink your milk!" is a refrain that has been heard throughout many a childhood. Today, with the availability of low-fat and nonfat milk, the one negative factor about milk—its high fat content—can be almost entirely eliminated.

Milk is an excellent source of calcium, riboflavin, vitamin D, vitamin B_{12}, and phosphorus; vitamin D is added back after pasteurization. Your body needs the combination of calcium, vitamin D, and phosphorus to build strong, healthy bones and teeth. In addition, calcium aids the blood in clotting, regulates hormones, assists the body in the absorption of vitamin B, and helps to maintain normal blood pressure and heart function.

Since your skeleton is essentially replaced every seven to ten years, it is extremely important to maintain proper calcium intake throughout your life. This is particularly important for women. During adolescence, pregnancy, lactation, and menopause and right after, women need a high calcium intake—1,200 milligrams a day. Women who consume less run an increased risk of osteoporosis—brittle, easily broken bones—in later life.

Drinking milk can be a problem for some people due to lactose intolerance, which is the inability to digest significant amounts of lactose, the predominant sugar in milk and many milk products. The inability is caused by a shortage of the digestive enzyme lactase. When your body doesn't produce enough of the enzyme to digest the lactose you consume, the result can be diarrhea, gas, bloating, nausea, and cramps. (Lactose intolerance is not the same as an allergy to cow's milk.) People vary in their degree of lactose intolerance. Some may find that they can tolerate a small glass of milk but not a large one; others can eat ice cream but cannot drink milk. In addition, your level of lactose intolerance can change over time, usually for the worse.

If you are lactose intolerant, avoid milk and milk products in the quantities that make you ill. You can still get the calcium, protein, B vitamins, and other benefits of milk by drinking the lactose-reduced milk and other products that are readily available in most supermarkets. Alternatively, you could purchase lactase tablets over the counter in a drugstore and add them to the milk yourself. Avoid raw milk, which does not contain less lactose—and since it's not pasteurized, drinking it could lead to illness. Acidophilus milk, although not dangerous, does not contain less lactose, either. Cultured buttermilk has slightly less lactose than what is in an equivalent amount of regular milk and may be tolerated a little better.

Because of consumer concerns about the fat content of milk, dairy producers now offer a range of milk with reduced fat. Here's how to tell them apart:

Whole milk. Still the most popular form of milk, whole milk contains at least 3.5 percent milk fat. Most recipes calling for milk mean whole milk, but in many cases, you can substitute lower-fat milk with little or no change in texture or flavor.

Two percent milk. Milk that has only 2 percent milk fat may be a better choice healthwise, but recent studies have shown that 2 percent milk is still far less healthy than the nonfat variety.

One percent milk. This version contains from 0.5 to 1 percent milk fat—a good step down on the fat scale from 2 percent milk, with just enough fat left to give it a richer color and taste than skim milk.

Skim or nonfat milk. Because this milk has less than 0.5 percent milk fat, it tends to have a watery consistency and bluish tinge.

Acidophilus milk. This is skim or low-fat milk that has acidophilus bacteria added to it. The bacteria are said to aid in digestion, but they will not help people who are lactose intolerant.

Lactose-reduced milk. This milk contains only 30 percent of the lactose in regular milk. Many people who aren't severely lactose intolerant can drink this milk in moderate quantities. If you are severely lactose intolerant, however, you will probably have to avoid it.

Cook's Note

To prevent spoilage, fresh milk must be kept refrigerated at 40 degrees F.

❖ Miso

A staple in Japanese cuisine, miso is the name given to both the soybean paste and to the clear soup made with the paste. Miso paste is made from fermented soybeans. It is quite salty and tastes a little like soy sauce; it resembles creamy peanut butter.

Because miso is made from soybeans, it contains phyto-estrogens, plant substances that are similar to the female hormone estrogen. Researchers believe that genistein, a compound found in soybeans and soy foods, may help protect women against breast cancer. Studies in Japan suggest that a daily bowl of miso soup can help protect against stomach cancer.

Miso is an excellent course of iron, B vitamins (including folate), and zinc. The high sodium content (over 5,000 milligrams in a 1/2-cup serving) is a drawback, however. Miso also contains tyramine, an amino acid derivative, that can trigger migraine headaches in those who are sensitive to it. Furthermore, if you take an MAO inhibiting drug (some antidepressants, for example), tyramine can raise your blood pressure.

❖ Mung Beans (Gram Beans or Mung Dal)

Small, round, green yellow or black beans with yellow flesh, mung beans are native to India and have been cultivated in China for millennia. In Asia, mung beans are eaten in many forms (cellophane noodles are made from mung bean flour), but in America, most mung beans are consumed as sprouts.

These delicate sprouts teem with nutritional goodness: protein, B vitamins (including large amounts of folate and thiamine), vitamin C, iron, magnesium, and potassium.

Cook's Note
Today, fresh mung bean sprouts are readily available at most grocery stores. Look for crisp, fresh sprouts with no signs of browning. Store fresh sprouts in a plastic bag in the refrigerator.

❖ Mushrooms

A culinary delight, beloved by epicures around the world, mushrooms come in an array of sizes, shapes, colors, and flavors. Different varieties of mushrooms provide different nutrients, but basically all are low in calories, fat-free, sodium-free, and supply a surprising amount of fiber. They also contain niacin, iron, and riboflavin, plus a number of other trace minerals. Shiitake mushrooms, a popular Japanese species, contain a substance called lentinan, which the Japanese use as a treatment for cancer. Recent studies suggest that lentinan stimulates the immune system, which may help the body to fight off cancer and viral infections. Extracts from the reishi mushroom, a less commonly known Asian species, may stop the growth of some tumors. Promising as the research is, you can't get the beneficial effects simply by eating lots of these mushrooms.

Numerous mushroom species are now commonly found in the produce section. Here are a few of the most popular:

Button mushrooms. This mild, white mushroom is the traditional classic.

Cèpe (porcini). These large, flavorful, firm-fleshed mushrooms are used in French and Italian cooking. They have a brownish color.

Chanterelles. With a flavor reminiscent of apricots, this slightly sweet mushroom has a yellow-orange cap.

Enoki. Tiny caps at the end of long, slender stems give these delicate, mild Oriental mushrooms a distinctive appearance.

Morels. Available in a wide vairety of sizes and colors ranging from dark brown to a creamy white, morels have conical, spongy, hollow caps. These mushrooms are beloved of French chefs and have a memorable scent and flavor. They are gathered wild.

Oyster mushrooms. These bluish-gray, mild mushrooms are often used in Asian cooking.

Shiitake. These large-capped, brown mushrooms are now familiar from Japanese cuisine. Shiitake mushrooms have a tough stem that is usually discarded before cooking.

Cook's Note

Dried mushrooms should be soaked in warm water (or a cooking liquid such as sherry) for about 15 minutes, or until they are soft. Three ounces of dried mushrooms are equivalent to 1 pound of fresh mushrooms.

❖ Mustard Greens

Pleasantly bitter in taste, mustard greens (a member of the cruciferous family of dark green, leafy vegetables) deliver a one-two punch of flavor and nutrition to your diet. A 1/2-cup serving of chopped, cooked mustard greens contains only 11 calories and just a trace of fat, but provides 30 percent of the RDA for vitamin C, 26 percent of the RDA for folate, 21 percent of the RDA for vitamin A, 6 percent of the RDA for calcium, and a bit of iron to boot. Add to that list the antioxidant compounds called indoles.

Cook's Note
Most mustard greens sold in the United States have bright green, oval, frilly-edged leaves with long stems. Some varieties range in color from light to dark green, and may have curly or smooth leaves. Mustard greens have a pungent, sharp taste something like prepared mustard. Swirl mustard greens gently in a large bowl of water, changing the water several times, to remove any grit clinging to the leaves. Cut out any blemished areas and remove tough stems.

❖ Nuts

Nuts have always been enjoyed as a snack food by themselves and as a crunchy, flavorful addition to other foods. As research reveals how valuable nuts can be for good health, they are becoming increasingly popular.

Nuts in general are good natural sources of vitamin E, thiamine, fiber, protein, and monounsaturated fat. They're also high in copper, a mineral that, according to some studies, may help keep you from feeling aches and pains. If you get frequent nonmigraine headaches, try adding a daily ounce or two of nuts to your diet. If you suffer from migraines, though, avoid nuts. They contain tyramine, a substance that is a common migraine trigger. Nuts are also a good source of the trace minerals boron and manganese, which help you metabolize calcium. Adding these minerals to your diet by eating a handful of nuts every day could help prevent or slow osteoporosis later in life. Hazelnuts, peanuts (technically a legume, not a nut), and almonds are especially high in boron; almonds also contain calcium. Brazil nuts are an excellent source of selenium, a trace mineral needed to make the antioxidant enzyme glutathione. All nuts are high in arginine, an amino acid that some herpes sufferers say worsens their symptoms. If you have herpes, avoiding nuts and peanuts may keep down the frequency of your outbreaks and the severity of the symptoms.

Cook's Note

Their high oil content means that nuts can become rancid if stored too long. Sniff nuts that have been stored for a while; if they are rancid, you'll be able to smell it. How can you tell if a nut in the shell is fresh? Shake it. If you hear the meat rattling around inside, the nut has become dry and stale.

See also Almonds; Brazil Nuts; Cashews; Hazelnuts; Peanuts; Pecans; Walnuts.

❖ Oats

Back in the good old days, before the advent of sugar-laden breakfast cereals and frozen waffles, many folks started the day with a big, steaming bowl of oatmeal. Unbeknownst to them, that soul-warming, belly-filling, chewy porridge was one of the healthiest meals going. Oats, either in the form of oatmeal or oat bran, have a remarkable ability to lower cholesterol levels in the blood. A number of studies have shown that people with a blood cholesterol level above 220 (considered high) can lower their total cholesterol level by 8 to 23 percent just by eating 3/4 cup of cooked oatmeal a day. For those at risk of developing heart disease, this is particularly good news, since every 1 percent drop in your cholesterol level lessens the risk of heart disease by 2 percent. For a while, researchers believed that it was the oat bran that did the trick, and that eating the bran alone would fight cholesterol even better. Recent studies, though, have shown that while oat bran is indeed higher in fiber (15 to 26 percent, compared to oatmeal's 7 percent), oatmeal is higher in polyunsaturated fatty acids, which have a cholesterol-lowering effect equal to fiber. Ideally, a healthy diet should include both.

Another benefit of oats is that they contain no gluten. This makes them a good food for people with celiac disease and wheat allergies. Oats can also help diabetics control their blood sugar levels.

A 3/4-cup serving of cooked oatmeal provides 4.6 grams of protein, 18.9 grams of carbohydrates, and 3.9 grams of dietary fiber, plus goodly amounts of thiamine, iron, magnesium, and zinc—all for 109 hunger-satisfying calories.

Oat bran is the outer casing of the oat kernel; it is sold in bulk in health food stores as a coarse meal and is also available as a breakfast cereal. Two tablespoons of oat bran provide 1.8 grams of dietary fiber, 2.0 grams of protein, and 7.7 grams of carbohydrates.

Other popular forms of oats include:

Oat groats. Check your health food store for oat groats, which are hulled, toasted oat kernels. This treatment allows groats to retain the most nutrition from the oat kernel. Use groats as you would rice—as a base for a casserole, as a side dish, or for stuffing, or cook and eat as you would oatmeal.

Steel-cut oats. Probably most familiar as Irish or Scotch oats, these are oat groats that have been coarsely cut. Because they are not flattened like oatmeal, steel-cut oats take longer to cook and have a distinctive chewy texture and rich, nutty flavor.

Old-fashioned rolled oats and quick-cooking rolled oats. The most familiar forms of oatmeal, these are oats that have been steamed and then rolled to flatten the kernels. Old-fashioned oats are whole, hulled grains that have been steamed and rolled flat; quick-cooking rolled oats are first chopped, then steamed and rolled to allow them to cook more quickly.

Instant oatmeal. Made from groats that have been pre-cooked and dried before rolling, instant oatmeal kernels are very soft and require only the addition of boiling water to be ready for eating. The main drawback of instant oatmeal is that it is available only in commercial packages to which sugar and salt are almost invariably added.

Oat flour. Flour can also be made from oats by processing the groats into a fine powder; you can also buy oat flour at health food stores. Use it to make muffins, quick breads, and cakes. If you are making yeast breads, combine it with wheat flour—otherwise, the bread won't rise, since oats contain no gluten.

Cook's Note

Some easy ways to add more oat power to your diet: Sprinkle oat bran over cereals, yogurt, or salads, substitute it for bread crumbs in recipes such as meat loaf, use it to bread fillets, or prepare it hot as a cereal. Oatmeal is wonderful in toppings for fruit cobblers or crisps and as an addition to vegetable soup, biscuits, muffins, cakes, and granola.

❖ Olives

The olive is actually a fruit. First cultivated in Greece, olives are now commercially produced in most Mediterranean countries. Within the United States, California has emerged as the leading producer. Raw olives are extremely bitter and must be cured to become edible. This curing is often done in brine (a salt solution) or soda; the process neutralizes and eventually removes the bitter taste.

Although olives are very high in oil (as you would assume), it is almost entirely the beneficial monounsaturated kind, which can actually help to control high cholesterol levels. Olives also contain a good amount of iron, and some protein and fiber. As an essential element in Mediterranean and Middle Eastern cooking, olives have a rich flavor that adds depth and piquancy to many dishes. More and more olive varieties are now readily available:

Black ripe olives. Cured to remove any bitterness, these olives are exposed to air during the rinsing process to give them a rich, dark brown to black color. Organic iron salt is added as a color fixative and the olives are canned in a brine solution. Drain and rinse before using.

Green ripe olives. These olives are cured in the same manner as black ripe olives, but they retain their natural green color because they are not exposed to air.

Spanish-style green olives. Fermented for four to six months in an acidic solution and packed in salt brine to add flavor, these green olives are often pitted and stuffed with red pimiento.

Sicilian-style olives. Medium green in color, these olives cured in salt brine are larger in size and have a crisp, salty flavor.

Greek-style olives. Usually made from olives that have been allowed to ripen fully on the tree, these are dry-salt cured, and rubbed with olive oil. A distinctive, strong taste and black, wrinkled appearance are the trademarks of Greek olives.

Kalamata (calamata). Another Greek-style olive, these are almond-shaped and purplish black in color. Kalamata olives are slit before being cured in brine and are packed in vinegar, giving them both a distinctive aroma and flavor.

Gaeta. A mild-flavored, Italian-style olive that is dry-salt cured, rubbed with olive oil, and usually packed with a variety of herbs, including rosemary.

Niçoise. France's contribution, this brown to dark brown green olive is small and very flavorful.

❖ Olive Oil

For years, doctors have noted that the levels of heart disease in the Mediterranean countries is surprisingly low. Recent studies suggest that olive oil, a central element in Mediterranean cuisine, may be part of the reason. The fat in olive oil is almost entirely monounsaturated, and many nutritionists believe that monounsaturated fat can help raise your blood levels of HDL (good) cholesterol. Adding olive oil to your diet, along with complex carbohydrates and fiber—the Mediterranean diet—could help to prevent coronary artery disease. The benefits come, however, only if you substitute olive oil for saturated fats (butter, margarine, oils, shortening, etc.) in your diet. Olive oil is becoming increasingly popular both for its healthful qualities and its subtle flavor. Three basic types are readily found in any supermarket:

Extra virgin. Unrefined, it has the richest flavor and lowest acidity of all the olive oils. Since it is the most costly of the olive oils, use extra virgin in small amounts as a flavor enhancer. Extra virgin oil is made from the first pressing of the olives and can range in color from dark green to gold.

Virgin. Also unrefined, this oil is less fruity and more acidic than extra virgin oil. The flavor can vary depending upon the producer. Virgin olive oil is made from first and second pressings; the color is usually a paler green or gold.

Olive oil or pure olive oil. This oil is made from unrefined virgin oil combined with refined oil. It is less flavorful but also less expensive.

❖ Onions

One of the world's oldest cultivated vegetables, onions (including leeks, shallots, scallions, and chives) are members of the lily family. They have been recommended as a healthful food for millennia. Indeed, the ancient Greek historian Herodotus advised the early Olympic athletes to eat onions to "lighten the balance of the blood." Interestingly, what the ancients recommended is being echoed by researchers today.

Few vegetables offer so much flavor and nutrition for so few calories. One medium onion (about 3 ounces or 150 grams) has just 60 calories and contains 2.8 grams of dietary fiber. It has only 10 milligrams of sodium but contains 200 milligrams of potassium. With nearly 12 milligrams of vitamin C, one medium onion provides 20 percent of the recommended daily allowance. Onions are also a good source for some of the B vitamins. A medium onion contains 120 micrograms or about 6 percent of the recommended daily allowance of vitamin B_6 (thiamine) and 24 micrograms or about 6 percent of the recommended daily allowance of folic acid (vitamin B_{12}). You can also get 38 milligrams of calcium (4 percent of the recommended daily allowance) from one onion.

In addition to high levels of dietary fiber, vitamins, and minerals, onions are the richest dietary source of quercetin, a powerful, naturally occurring antioxidant compound. Preliminary studies suggest that quercetin may work to help prevent cancer cells and blood clots from forming, help inhibit allergic and inflammatory responses, and help stop infections. Onions also seem to have blood-thinning abilities because they contain adenosine, a naturally occurring chemical that has been shown to help lower LDL (bad) cholesterol in the blood and to lower blood pressure. Adenosine also plays an important role in inhibiting blood clots. The prostaglandins A1 and E, which play a role in naturally lowering blood pressure, have also been isolated from onions. It's no surprise, then, that cardiologists frequently advise heart patients to eat raw onions to help increase blood circulation, lower blood pressure, and reduce the chances of dangerous blood clots.

A major study in China sponsored by the National Cancer Institute showed that eating garlic and onions protects against stomach cancer. People in Shandong Province who ate 3 ounces of garlic and onions daily had far lower rates of stomach cancer than those who ate less. In all probability, the sulfur compounds and quercetin in onions are responsible for the protective effect. The powerful anti-inflammatory effects of the quercetin in onions has also been shown to help asthma sufferers reduce the number and severity of their attacks.

All in all, it's probably a good idea to add onions to your diet. Here's a list of the most popular varieties:

Yellow onions. Smallish to large, yellow in color, and strong in flavor, traditional yellow onions are the most common and least expensive variety.

Sweet onions. These onions, including the Bermuda, Maui, Sweet Vidalia, Jumbo Spanish, and Walla Walla varieties, are juicy and sweet enough to eat out of hand. They range in color from ivory to light brown. Many sweet onion varieties are seasonal and available only in the spring and summer.

Red onions. A spicy-sweet taste distinguishes these colorful onions, but they do not hold up to long cooking. Use them to add color, crunch, and flavor to salads, on sandwiches and burgers, or in quick-cooking dishes.

White boiling onions. Small and mild, these onions are most often added to stews and soups or are creamed for a side dish.

Cook's Note

Select onions that are firm to the touch, with dry, clean skins, and no soft spots or green sprouts. Most onion varieties should be stored in a cool, dark place.

❖ Oranges

One orange gives you more than a full day's RDA of vitamin C. That alone would be enough to make oranges a valuable food for good health. In addition, however, oranges also offer fiber, flavonoids (some of which are antioxidants), and terpene; these help limit your body's production of cholesterol and help produce enzymes that could deactivate certain carcinogens. In particular, studies have shown that people who eat a lot of oranges have lower rates of pancreatic cancer. The flavonoids and vitamin C work together to help strengthen your immune system and support the connective tissues in your body. Iron, potassium, magnesium, niacin, and riboflavin are thrown in for good measure.

Native to China and Southeast Asia, oranges are now cultivated worldwide. California and Florida produce most of the oranges grown in the United States. Other citrus fruits, including citrons, mandarin oranges, tangerines, and tangelos, provide benefits similar to oranges.

See also Grapefruit.

❖ Papayas

A mildly sweet, pear-shaped tropical fruit, papayas can grow up to 20 inches long. The papaya is an even better dietary source of vitamin C than an orange: a 1/2-cup serving yields an amazing 157 percent of the RDA. Papaya also contains generous amounts of folate and beta carotene. Like most fruits, papaya supplies an abundant amount of fiber (2.6 grams in a 1/2-cup serving).

Papaya is a traditional Caribbean remedy for indigestion and stomach ailments. There's a scientific basis for this, since papaya contains an enzyme called papain that aids in the digestion of protein.

Cook's Note

Thanks to refrigeration, you can enjoy papayas year round. You can't eat the greenish yellow skin, but the golden orange flesh can be eaten raw or cooked. The juice can be enjoyed as a chilled drink. The seeds can also be eaten or used as a garnish.

❖ Parsley

The sprig of parsley that typically decorates a dinner plate is definitely good enough to eat. This leafy green is rich in vitamin C, folate, iron, and vitamin A—and it even freshens your breath. Furthermore, parsley is a member of the umbelliferous vegetable family, which also includes carrots, celery, dill, fennel, parsnips, and caraway. These vegetables are currently being studied by researchers at the National Cancer Institute and elsewhere because they contain so many cancer-fighting compounds.

In addition to the obvious benefits of this vitamin-rich plant, parsley has several lesser-known properties. Parsley contains chlorophyll, vitamin C, flavonoids, and carotenes. Natural medicine practitioners often recommend eating parsley if you are taking the antibiotic drug tetracycline. They claim the parsley helps offset the vitamin C depletion that may occur with this drug. Tea made from parsley is said to help relieve the symptoms of the common cold and to act as a mild diuretic; some say it is also good for digestion. For a natural breath freshener, try chewing on fresh parsley sprigs.

❖ Parsnips

Another member of the illustrious umbelliferous vegetable family, parsnips are kin to carrots, parsley, and celery. Of Mediterranean origin, this winter root vegetable has a sweet and nutty flavor when cooked. In the nutrition department, a 1/2-cup serving of parsnips provides 3.8 grams of dietary fiber, 23 percent of the RDA for folate, and a whopping 15.2 grams of complex carbohydrates—for only 63 calories. All this makes parsnips a healthful, hearty addition to a meal and a boon to those trying to control their weight.

Today, much interest is focused on the ability of parsnips and other members of the umbelliferous vegetable family to fight cancer. All these vegetables, parsnips included, contain phytochemicals such as terpene, which seem to play a role in protecting against tumors. They also contain plentiful amounts of vitamin C, an antioxidant.

Cook's Note
When shopping for parsnips, select smooth, firm, small to medium-sized roots. Avoid large parsnips—they may be woody and bitter.

❖ Peaches and Nectarines

Juicy, delectable peaches are low in calories (one medium-sized peach has only about 40) and are a good source of complex carbohydrates and fiber. In addition to vitamin C, boron, and potassium, peaches are rich in beta carotene. A fuzz-free relative of peaches, nectarines are nutritionally very similar to peaches, with an added helping of niacin.

Cook's Note

Peaches and nectarines both are at their peak during the late summer months, though they are available from late spring through the fall. A perfect peach should be plump and firm yet yield to gentle pressure, it should have a fuzzy, soft yellow to orange skin with patches of blush and no green. It should have no mushy, bruised, or sticky spots. There are two basic varieties of peaches: freestone and clingstone. Freestone peaches allow the flesh to be easily pulled away from the pit; clingstone, as the name implies, clings to the pit. To remove the skins from ripe peaches and nectarines, plunge them first into boiling water for 30 seconds, then plunge them into a bowl of ice water. The skin should slip right off.

❖ Peanuts

Not a nut at all, peanuts are actually legumes, members of the bean family. In the form of peanut butter, they are a favorite in sandwiches; roasted peanuts, in or out of the shell, are a favorite snack food. A 1-ounce serving of dry-roasted peanuts contains 164 calories and 14 grams of fat. Fortunately, most of this fat is the monounsaturated or polyunsaturated kind. Rich in folate, niacin, and other B vitamins, peanuts also offer a generous amount of dietary fiber (2.6 grams in a 1-ounce serving) and are a good source of magnesium and boron. Studies suggest that, like real nuts, peanuts can help protect you against heart disease.

Peanuts and peanut butter can be a source of aflatoxin, a naturally occurring, very potent carcinogen. Manufacturers of peanut products follow very stringent FDA guidelines to keep the amount of aflatoxin in their products to no more than 20 parts per billion—an amount that is extremely unlikely to have any toxic effects. To be on the safe side, however, be wary about purchasing "natural" peanut butter and other peanut products that may not have been produced under strict supervision. Keep peanut butter and other peanut products in a cool, dry place. Don't use them if they smell rancid, off, or are past their expiration date. Peanuts are also a fairly common food allergen, especially for children. Introduce peanuts slowly to young children and watch carefully for reactions.

If you have kidney stones, avoid peanuts—they are high in oxalate, which can contribute to stone formation. Peanuts are high in the amino acid arginine, which may cause flare-ups if you have herpes.

❖ Pears

One of the few fruits that ripens well after picking, pears contain large amounts of soluble fiber in the form of pectin. Actually, pears are even higher in pectin than apples. This plethora of pectin (and other soluble fiber) makes pears a terrific choice for helping to lower blood cholesterol levels and insuring the health of the digestive system. Pears also have a particularly good sodium-to-potassium ratio, which makes them a good snack if you have high blood pressure.

A single (6-ounce) pear provides 98 calories, 25.1 grams of complex carbohydrates, and 11 percent of the RDA for vitamin C. Dried pears offer many of the same nutritional pluses of fresh pears. Like all dried fruits, however, dried pears also concentrate the sugars and thus are considerably higher in calories.

Some fresh pears are sold in supermarkets virtually year round, but for the juiciest, most flavorful fruit, buy pear varieties when they are in season. Some of the most popular varieties are:

Anjou. Yellow green in color, plump, and large in size, this all-purpose dessert pear is quite juicy when ripe. The delicate, winey flavor is best displayed in dishes that don't overwhelm it with spices. In season from October to April.

Bartlett. Red or yellow in color with a bare hint of green, these firm-fleshed pears have a definitive pear taste. Bartlett pears stand up well to cooking and are ideal for canning. In season from July to mid-October.

Bosc. Russet red, long-necked, and large in size, Bosc pears have an intense flavor with slightly spicy undertones. Fragrant and crisp, these pears lend themselves to baking, poaching, and sautéing. In season from October to February.

Comice. Golden-skinned with a rosy blush, these fragile pears sometimes have surface blemishes, but they do not detract at all from the fragrant, buttery flesh. Comice pears are probably the sweetest and juiciest of the larger pears, and are best eaten fresh and uncooked. In season from October through March.

Seckel. A variety of Comice pears, Seckels are often used in condiments and as garnishes. These petite pears, sometimes called sugar pears, have a rich, spicy flavor. In season from late August to December.

❖ Peas

Peas are a potent source of a number of vitamins and minerals, including folate, vitamin C, thiamine, iron, magnesium, niacin, vitamin B_6, riboflavin, potassium, and zinc. A 1/2-cup serving of fresh, boiled green peas provides 4.3 grams of protein, 12.5 grams of complex carbohydrates, and 2.4 grams of insoluble dietary fiber—for only 67 calories and virtually no fat. Like their fresh cousins, dried peas (whole or split, yellow or green) are an excellent source of vegetable protein, complex carbohydrates, and fiber.

Cook's Note

When using fresh or frozen peas in soups and stews, add them at the end of the recipe so they don't get mushy. Use dried peas in soups and stews. Dried and split peas do not need to be soaked before using.

❖ Pecans

Related to the hickory, pecan trees can grow to 180 feet, though most are in the 75- to 90-foot range. An American original, pecans are native to the Mississippi River valleys. The United States is not only the primary producer of pecans, it is practically the *only* producer.

Like most nuts, pecans are full of dietary fiber (1.9 grams in a 1-ounce serving). They are also high in fat (91 percent of the calories comes from fat), though most of this is the monounsaturated variety, which can actually help lower blood cholesterol levels. Particularly rich in thiamine, magnesium, and zinc, pecans also contain folic acid and iron.

See also Nuts.

❖ Peppers (Sweet Peppers or Bell Peppers)

In season year round, peppers (also called sweet peppers or bell peppers) come in a veritable rainbow of colors: green, red, yellow, orange, purple, and gold. Spicy sweet in flavor, peppers can be used raw or cooked. In addition to color, they add a whopping dose of vitamin C to any dish. Since all peppers are part of the same family, the only difference between these peppers and hot peppers is the hotness.

A 1/2-cup serving of chopped pepper (about half a medium-sized pepper) has only 14 calories but provides 74 percent of the RDA of vitamin C. Folate and vitamin B_6 are also present in good amounts. Sweet red peppers contain even more vitamin C than their green counterparts: 158 percent of the RDA in a 1/2-cup serving, plus a generous amount of beta carotene and an antioxidant carotenoid called lycopene. Studies suggest that people with low lycopene levels have a higher risk of cervical, bladder, and pancreatic cancers.

See also Hot Peppers.

❖ Pineapple

The ultimate taste of the tropics, just the scent of fresh pineapple brings to mind long walks on white sand beaches, with palm trees swaying in a warm breeze. Although satisfyingly sweet, pineapple won't spoil the way you look in a bathing suit—1 cup of fresh pineapple cubes contains only 76 calories; a cup of canned pineapple chunks in unsweetened pineapple juice has 140 calories. While not the powerhouse of nutrition that some fruits are, pineapple offers a good array of vitamins and minerals, including thiamine, folate, vitamin B_6, iron, and magnesium, plus a decent dose of vitamin C (40 percent of the RDA in a 1-cup serving). Pineapple also contains bromelain, a protein-digesting enzyme, which can aid digestion and help relieve inflammation. But pineapple's real value comes from its high manganese content. This mineral is essential for building and maintaining healthy bones and helping to prevent osteoporosis. In addition, women with very heavy menstrual flows often have low levels of manganese; when manganese is added to their diets, their flows diminish.

Cook's Note

Select a ripe pineapple by its heady aroma. Look for one that is heavy for its size, with flesh that yields when gently pressed. The easiest way to cut up a fresh pineapple is to cut it in half lengthwise from the stem through the leafy crown. Cut each pineapple half in half again lengthwise. Using a thin-bladed knife, cut the flesh from each pineapple quarter in one large piece. Hold each quarter on end and slice off and discard the tough core. Cut each cored quarter lengthwise in half, then slice across into chunks.

❖ Plantains

Botanically a fruit, plantains are usually treated as a starchy vegetable and used as a side dish. Plantains look like huge bananas (a close relative), but have thicker skins, are tougher, more starchy, and cannot be eaten raw. Unripe green plantains are bland in taste and are most often boiled and mashed, fried, or used in soups and stews; ripe plantains are yellow to brown in color, sweeter in taste (somewhat like sweet potatoes) and are suited to baking or sautéing. When the skin of a plantain turns black, it is fully ripe, very sweet (like bananas), and perfect for serving as a sweet side dish or stewing for dessert.

A 1/2-cup serving of cooked plantain slices registers a low 89 calories with 0.1 grams of fat, no cholesterol, and 24 grams of complex carbohydrates. With 1.8 grams of fiber in the same serving, plantains can definitely help keep the digestive system in good working order. Plantains also contain vitamin A, vitamin B_6, vitamin C, folic acid, magnesium, potassium, and sodium.

❖ Potatoes

Potatoes are native to the Andes region of Bolivia and Peru, where they have been cultivated for over 7,000 years. Potatoes were introduced to Europe and the rest of the world in the 1700s, and they quickly became a staple food. Filling, delicious, easy to grow, inexpensive, and very nutritious, the potato is now used in cuisines the world over.

Practically perfect in every way, the potato offers an amazing array of nutritional benefits. A single 7-ounce baked potato with skin has 844.4 milligrams of potassium—over twice that of a banana—28 percent of the RDA for iron, 43 percent of the RDA for vitamin C, and 35 percent of the RDA for vitamin B_6, plus generous amounts of niacin, magnesium, thiamine, and folate. Furthermore, the same potato contains 51 grams of complex carbohydrates, 4.7 grams of protein (including lysine, an amino acid generally missing in vegetable protein sources), 2.2 grams of dietary fiber, and just 220 calories, only 1 percent of which are from fat.

Plain potatoes—boiled, baked, or mashed—are a good choice if you have mild diarrhea or an upset stomach. Plain potatoes are bland and easy to digest, and the starchiness can help relieve diarrhea.

Cook's Note

Select firm, smooth, unblemished potatoes that are heavy for their size. Avoid potatoes that have sprouted, are mushy, or have green patches. The green can indicate the presence of solanine, an alkaloid that is mildly toxic.

Resist the urge to smother potatoes in fatty butter or sour cream or to deep-fry them. Instead, try topping baked potatoes with fat-free sour cream or, better yet, nonfat yogurt. And always eat the skins—much of the nutrition is near the surface.

❖ Prunes and Prune Juice

Prunes are one of nature's richest sources of dietary fiber. A single serving of six prunes (about 1/4 cup) has just 110 calories and almost 3 grams of dietary fiber (nearly 10 percent of the recommended daily value). This fiber consists mostly of a soluble type called pectin. A serving of prunes has virtually no sodium, but does contain close to 300 milligrams of potassium (about 8 percent of the RDA). It also contains about 10 percent of the RDA for vitamin A. Prune juice provides most of the nutrients and fiber of dried prunes. Bottled prune juice is an all-natural product with no added sugar.

The low calories and sweet taste of prunes have traditionally made them a favorite source of dietary fiber. Doctors often recommend a daily serving of prunes to treat constipation and promote regularity. Patients with painful hemorrhoids usually find that a daily serving of prunes helps them have less painful bowel movements. Why are prunes such a good laxative? No one really knows, although researchers suspect the answer may lie in the laxative effect of the sorbitol. On the other hand, since sorbitol can cause a flare-up of symptoms for people with irritable bowel syndrome, sufferers should avoid prunes and other high-sorbitol foods, such as apple juice, pears, and sorbitol-sweetened diet foods.

Prunes and prune juice are also valuable for pregnant and nursing women. During pregnancy, women need additional fluids to aid in carrying nutrients through the body, and nursing women need extra fluids to aid in producing milk.

Prune juice is a satisfying and nutritious choice. The high potassium content of prunes and prune juice helps women metabolize salt better and helps prevent water retention during pregnancy and while nursing.

Cook's Note

Prunes are unique in their high levels of naturally occurring pectins, sorbitol (a natural sugar), and malic acid (a natural preservative). Because these ingredients naturally add flavor, texture, and moistness, prunes can be used instead of shortening in muffins, brownies, cookies, and other bakery treats. Substituting pureed prunes or prepared prune butter for butter, margarine, or oil can slash the fat content by 75 to 90 percent without sacrificing taste.

❖ Pumpkin

For most people, this hardy winter squash makes its dietary appearance as pie once a year at Thanksgiving, but pumpkin is a nutritious and versatile food that deserves more of our attention. Pumpkin is an outstanding source of beta carotene—over 250 percent of the RDA for vitamin A is found in just 1/2 cup of mashed pumpkin. Pumpkin also provides ample rations of fiber and iron, and a good measure of vitamin C, folic acid, magnesium, potassium, complex carbohydrates, and protein as well. All these health benefits from 1/2 cup add up to only 41 calories. Canned pumpkin puree offers the same nutrients as fresh pumpkin in a more convenient, year-round form.

Pumpkin seeds are loaded with a wide array of vitamins and minerals (including zinc) and have a high content of essential amino acids. Some evidence suggests that amino acids, including alanine, glycine, and glutamine, can help relieve the symptoms of benign prostate enlargement.

❖ Purslane

A sturdy green resembling clover, purslane is widely regarded as a weed. This weed, however, packs a nutritional wallop, and health-conscious cooks are now adding purslane to salads. With a nutty flavor and a texture somewhat like bean sprouts, purslane is a terrific source of vitamins A, C, and E, magnesium, potassium, calcium, and large amounts of omega-3 fatty acids, which can help lower your blood cholesterol levels.

Cook's Note
Wash purslane well and toss it in a green salad, add it to stews and soups, both as a thickening agent and to add flavor, or just steam or sauté it lightly (like spinach) and serve as a side dish.

❖ Quinoa

An ancient "grain" originally found in the Andes region of Peru and Bolivia, quinoa (pronounced *keen-wa* or *kee-no-ah*) is actually the fruit of an herb. In appearance, quinoa is similar to sesame seeds: small, round, off-white kernels. The seeds can be cooked and served like rice, but they take only 20 minutes to cook. The flavor of quinoa is quite mild, which makes it a good base for seasoned vegetable or meat dishes. Quinoa can also be served as a side dish, used in casseroles, added to a salad, or used as the base of a dessert similar to rice pudding.

This rediscovered grain is a veritable treasure trove of nutrition—no wonder the Incas referred to it as the "mother grain." Quinoa's amino acid content makes it one of the best nonanimal sources of protein now available. A 1/2-cup serving of cooked quinoa is about 129 calories, yet contains all eight of the essential amino acids necessary to make a complete protein. This is unusual, because generally, complete proteins are found only in foods from animal sources: meat, dairy products, and eggs. Of the three amino acids found in grains—lysine, methionine, and cysteine—quinoa offers even more than most actual grains do. Quinoa is low in fat and is an excellent source of both dietary fiber and complex carbohydrates. Rich in magnesium and potassium, quinoa also supplies good amounts of iron, folate, riboflavin, zinc, and niacin.

Cook's Note

Until recently, quinoa was only available at natural or health food stores, but more and more supermarkets are packaging and selling quinoa. Rinse raw quinoa well before using, as the outer coating is quite bitter.

❖ Radishes

Radishes, like parsley, are often relegated to the position of garnish, without consideration of their nutritional benefits. The radish is actually a valuable member of the famous cruciferous family of cancer-fighting vegetables. A 1/2-cup serving of sliced radishes has just 10 calories, but offers 1.2 grams of dietary fiber and is an excellent source of vitamin C and folate.

Aside from their nutritional value, radishes add refreshing sharpness and color to salads. A surprising range of varieties is available.

Black. Pungent and spicy, these radishes are black on the outside and creamy white on the inside.

Daikon. A Japanese radish, daikons are long and white with a mildly spicy flavor. Daikons may be served as you would turnips: raw, sliced, or cooked.

French breakfast radishes. The color of red radishes, the French breakfast variety has an elongated shape similar to icicle radishes.

Icicle. As the name implies, mild-flavored icicle radishes are white with an elongated shape.

Red. The most familiar radish is bright red on the outside and very white on the inside. Red radishes can range in flavor from quite mild to rather spicy.

Cook's Note

Purchase firm, brightly colored radishes; look for unblemished skins with no cracks or spots. Store fresh radishes in a plastic bag, refrigerated, for about a week. Try substituting fresh radishes for water chestnuts in Chinese cooking.

❖ Raisins

The modern parent's favorite take-along snack for their young, raisins are a terrific source of iron. They are also one of the few fruits that can be dried without adding the chemicals used in sulfurizing (a preserving process). Most of the commercially dried raisins found in the United States are made from Thompson seedless grapes. Like wine, the color of the raisin does not necessarily indicate the color of the grape when the process started. It is the drying process used that determines the final color of the raisin.

Golden seedless raisins and dark seedless raisins are quite similar in nutritional value. A 1/2-cup serving of either type contains about 218 calories. The same serving offers from 13 to 15 percent of the RDA for iron (you'll absorb more of the iron if you eat raisins along with a food rich in vitamin C, such as orange juice). Vitamin B_6, riboflavin, thiamine, and magnesium are also present in raisins, as is a liberal dose of dietary fiber. Raisins are also a valuable source of the mineral boron, essential for strong bones and for preventing osteoporosis.

Many pediatricians warn against giving raisins to children under the age of four for fear of choking.

❖ Rhubarb

The fibrous, pink-to-red stalks of rhubarb are thought to be native to northwest China and Tibet. The plant has been used there medicinally for over 2,000 years. The top, leafy portion of rhubarb contains a toxic amount of oxalate and should never be eaten.

The stalk has some nutritional value, but it is so tart that it must be mixed with sweeteners to make it palatable. It is high in calcium, but the mineral is in the form of calcium oxalate, which actually blocks the absorption of calcium by the body. The oxalate is also a hazard for people with kidney stones. Rhubarb is traditionally recommended as a laxative. In fact, a powdered form of the Chinese root is a very powerful purgative, but the stalks found in the supermarket or grown in the garden have virtually no laxative effect. Rhubarb can range in color from pale green with pinkish overtones to a deep red. Generally, the redder the stalk, the sweeter it is.

❖ Rice

The most popular grain in the world, rice is eaten as a staple food by more people in more countries than any other single grain. Most of the rice consumed, however, is polished white rice, which has been processed to strip off the husk, bran, and germ. Unfortunately, this process also removes about half of the rice's nutritional value. But for those who are devoted to white rice, there is another option: enriched white rice, or rice that has been sprayed with a solution containing various nutrients lost in the polishing process, then sealed with an edible coating. Other white rice types include converted or parboiled white rice, in which the grain is steamed and processed while the hull is still in place, forcing some of the nutrients into the core of the rice, and instant or precooked white rice, which is either partially or completely cooked, then dehydrated. As the name implies, instant rice cooks in a fraction of the time it takes to cook other rice, but both the texture and the nutrient value is diminished.

Brown rice has had only the inedible hull of the grain removed. The light brown color, chewy texture, and nutty flavor all make brown rice an appetizing option, though the slow cooking time makes this rice somewhat less convenient than white varieties. A 1/2-cup serving of cooked brown rice contains 110 calories, 23 grams of complex carbohydrates, 1.7 grams of dietary fiber, and 2.3 grams of protein. Brown rice is an excellent source of magnesium and offers good amounts of vitamin B_6, niacin, thiamine, and iron. Brown rice comes in long-, medium-, and short-grained varieties.

Half a cup of cooked white enriched rice, in comparison, has 133 calories, 29.2 grams of complex carbohydrates, 0.2 grams of dietary fiber, and 2.4 grams of protein. Because it has been sprayed with a nutrient solution, enriched white rice actually provides greater amounts of iron, thiamine, and niacin than brown rice, but its fiber content is very low because the bran has been removed.

Rice is starchy and easy to digest, which makes it an excellent food if you have diarrhea, heartburn, or an upset stomach. Rice is also a good choice if you have irritable bowel syndrome, celiac disease, or allergies to other grains such as wheat or corn. Rice bran (sold in health food stores) can help relieve constipation and could help reduce blood cholesterol levels.

Until recently, white rice was the predominant rice in the United States; brown rice was seen as a food primarily for "health-food nuts." Times change, however, and now brown rice is sold in every supermarket, along with a number of other varieties.

Long-grain rice. These grains are four to five times as long as they are wide. Available in both brown and white varieties, long-grain rice is fluffy when cooked; the grains separate easily.

Medium-grain rice. These grains are shorter in length and wider around than long-grain varieties. When cooked, medium-grain rice is fluffy yet tends to become somewhat sticky as it cools.

Short-grain rice. These grains are even shorter than medium-grain rice. Short-grain rice is particularly popular in China and Japan because it is soft and sticky when cooked—perfect for eating with chopsticks.

Arborio rice. A medium- to short-grain rice grown in Italy, this is the rice of choice for risotto. It has a rich, nutty flavor.

Aromatic rice. This category includes basmati (a long-grain white rice often used in Indian and Pakistani dishes) and texmati (a rice similar to basmati, available in both brown and white varieties). Aromatic rice is notable for its wonderful aroma, which has nutty or popcornlike overtones.

Sweet, glutinous, sticky, or waxy rice. This short-grain rice is very sticky when cooked, with a somewhat sweet flavor. It is particularly popular in Asian dishes.

Wild rice. This is actually a very dark purple grain from a grass grown primarily in the Great Lakes region of North America; however, wild rice does look like true rice when cooked. Chewy wild rice is often paired with white rice to great effect.

❖ Rye

Most familiar to Americans in flour form, rye flour makes a moist, richly flavored bread that is perfect for sandwiches. Rye flour also offers a range of nutrients that is more extensive than other grains. For example, 1/4 cup of rye flour contains 6.1 grams of dietary fiber. It also contributes a generous amount of protein, magnesium, folate, iron, niacin, and zinc, plus good amounts of thiamine, riboflavin, vitamin B_6, and vitamin E. Products made with rye flour tend to make the stomach feel full, so there is less chance of overeating (weight-watchers often swear by rye crackers as a diet aid).

Cook's Note
Sniff rye flour carefully before buying or using it, and don't use the flour if it smells musty. Rye can grow a mold called ergot, which if consumed can cause all manner of strange symptoms (one of the alkaloids present in ergot is lysergic acid diethylamide, known familiarly as LSD). When baking with rye flour, mix in an equal amount of wheat flour. On its own, rye doesn't have enough gluten to develop the necessary eleasticity for good bread.

❖ Seaweed

While not yet a staple of the American diet, seaweed is used in many Asian cuisines, notably Japanese, and its many health benefits may encourage a greater consumption throughout the rest of the world. There are a wide variety of seaweeds used for culinary purposes, and each has its own unique taste and nutritional advantage. Kelp, one of the most familiar seaweeds, has no fat, no cholesterol, is extremely low in calories, and provides generous amounts of folate, iodine (essential for your thyroid gland, but a possible cause of acne flare-ups in some people), magnesium, and, in smaller amounts, calcium and iron. Fresh kelp can be added to soup stocks for color and flavor; dried kelp (known as kombu) is used to wrap sushi and can be brewed as a tea. Other forms of edible seaweed include carrageenan, which is thought to prevent ulcers and blood clots; laminaria, which may help prevent high blood pressure and hardening of the arteries; hijiki or hiziki, a good source of dietary fiber, potassium, magnesium, riboflavin, and calcium; wakame, whose nutrient breakdown is similar to hijiki; and arame, which provides generous amounts of fiber, vitamin A, zinc, and calcium.

❖ Sesame Seeds

The seeds of the sesame plant have been harvested for centuries, both for the seeds themselves and for the oil made from them. And while most of the calories found in sesame seeds come from fat, almost all of the fat is in the form of monounsaturated and polyunsaturated oils, which can help in the fight against high blood cholesterol. One tablespoon of hulled sesame seeds (the hull is quite bitter and is usually removed) provides 8 percent of the RDA for magnesium, 6 percent of the RDA for iron, and 5 percent of the RDA for zinc. Sesamin, a type of fiber found only in sesame seeds, is thought to help lower blood cholesterol levels by lowering the absorption of cholesterol from the diet. Sesamin may also have an antioxidant effect.

Cook's Note
Toasting sesame seeds in a dry skillet over low heat until they are golden and fragrant brings out their full, nutty essence.

❖ Soybeans

From ancient China to contemporary society, the soybean is one of the oldest and most scrutinized food sources. Available as beans, sprouts, milk, paste, and in a host of other foods made with soy-based meal, this legume has economic, environmental, and nutritional advantages that raise it high above other beans and peas. Since one acre of soybeans can offer almost 20 percent of the protein that beef raised on the same acre could, soybeans are a terrifically economic crop. And the health benefits of soybeans and soy products are still being discovered.

A 1/2-cup serving of boiled soybeans offers 14.3 grams of protein—nearly twice that of other legumes—for a mere 149 calories and no cholesterol. The protein found in soybeans is very high quality, basically on the same level as animal protein, but without the fat and cholesterol. In fact, the protein in soybeans appears to actually help decrease the blood cholesterol level in the body, particularly for people whose cholesterol levels are very high. (Since the beneficial effect comes from the protein, eating soy sauce or soybean oil won't help.) Soybeans also contain high amounts of the animo acid lysine, which can help relieve the symptoms and severity of cold sores and herpes outbreaks. A serving of soybeans also provides 44 percent of the RDA for iron, 23 percent of the RDA for folate, and 21 percent of the RDA for magnesium, plus beneficial amounts of potassium, calcium, vitamin B_6, thiamine, and zinc. Soybeans do contain about 18 percent fat, most of which is monounsaturated. Some research suggests that a diet rich in soybeans or soybean-based foods may protect you against cancer. One reason for this is that soybeans are the best dietary source of protease inhibitors, which can help prevent cancer of the stomach, colon, liver, lung, pancreas, and esophagus. Recent studies have found that soybeans can stimulate the production of estrogen, which can be beneficial to menopausal and postmenopausal women. Paradoxically, the same phytoestrogens found in soy protein may also protect against some hormone-related cancers of the breast and prostate. One word of caution: Despite all of the wonderful and varied benefits soybeans offer, they are also a common food allergen. Check labels carefully if you are allergic to this food.

Soybeans can be incorporated into the diet in many ways. The dried beans require very long soaking and cooking to be palatable. Use dried beans in soups and stews. Soybeans are also the main ingredient in textured vegetable protein (TVP), a meat substitute sold in health food stores. An Indonesian specialty, tempeh, is a cake made from fermented soybeans. Soybeans are also used in miso and to make soy milk and tofu (bean curd).

See also Miso; Soy Milk; Tofu (Bean Curd).

❖ Soy Milk

Once limited to baby formulas and a few health food fans, soy milk has become increasingly popular in the past few years. A number of commercial brands are now readily available in natural food stores and even supermarkets. Soy milk is traditionally made by soaking soybeans in water, pulverizing the wet beans, and straining the remaining liquid. Because the natural flavor of soy milk is quite bland, commercial brands often add vanilla, chocolate, carob, or other flavorings to make a refreshing drink. Soy milk is also used to make a variety of frozen desserts that are a lower-fat alternative to their cream- and milk-based counterparts.

A boon to people who are lactose intolerant and can't drink cow's milk, soy milk is also beneficial for children who are allergic to milk. It is an excellent source of protein and provides virtually all the same benefits as soybeans themselves.

See also Soybeans.

❖ Spinach

Everyone knows that spinach is good for you, although they may be slightly misled as to why. The popular conception is that spinach is a good dietary source of iron, but it's actually the antioxidant beta carotenes in spinach that make this leafy green so valuable. Half a cup of steamed spinach has 74 percent of the RDA for vitamin A. You also get 66 percent of your daily folic acid and 15 percent of your daily calcium, and lots of fiber, for just 21 calories. Of course, spinach does contain a lot of iron, although much of it is in a form that can't be readily absorbed by your body. It also contains manganese, which is necessary for strong bones. Spinach is a good source of lutein, another potent antioxidant. In addition to helping to protect you against cancer, there's some evidence that the high levels of folic acid, beta carotene, lutein, and other antioxidants in spinach can also help keep cataracts from forming in the elderly. If you have a tendency toward kidney stones, however, the high oxalate content of spinach could cause you to form more stones.

Cook's Note

Fresh spinach must be washed thoroughly. Swirl it gently in a bowl of cool water. You'll probably have to rinse the spinach and change the water several times to get all the grit out. Spinach is delicious raw. Never overcook spinach— steam or sauté it very lightly. To help your body absorb more of the iron in spinach, add a dash of lemon juice, citrus sections, or red onions.

❖ Squash

A change of seasons means a change of squash, which comes in winter or summer varieties. Winter squash, such as pumpkin, have tough rinds, soft flesh, and an abundance of seeds. Summer squash have thin skins, delicate flesh, and edible seeds. The ubiquitous zucchini is the most common and popular summer squash. Although their nutritional values differ, all these squashes are part of the same healthy family.

Summer squash varieties include zucchini, yellow, and pattypan. All are best eaten when young, firm, and very fresh. A dieter's delight, summer squash is extremely low in calories (a 1/2-cup serving of steamed zucchini has only 14 calories). These squash are good sources of beta carotene and vitamin C.

The tough, durable rinds of winter squash mean they can be stored without refrigeration for long periods of time. The yellow or orange color of their flesh is a clue to their primary nutritional value: these squash are loaded with antioxidant beta carotenes. Study after study indicates that eating these squash on a regular basis can help protect you against heart disease, cancer, cataracts, and other ailments. Popular varieties of winter squash include:

Acorn. This squash has a dark green rind with orange markings and is shaped, as the name suggests, like an acorn. The golden orange flesh tastes slightly sweet and nutty.

Buttercup. A dark green rind with gray spots and a shape a bit like a turban characterize this squash. It has a smooth, sweet-tasting flesh, though it is somewhat drier than other winter squashes.

Butternut. Shaped like a gourd with a long neck and round bottom, butternut squash is pale golden in color and has a buttery taste to its yellow orange flesh.

Golden Nugget. Small (about the size of an apple) and bright golden orange in color, this squash resembles nothing so much as a miniature pumpkin.

Hubbard. With a rind that can appear greenish gray, bluish green, or orange in color, Hubbard squashes are very large with a ridged rind. Often sold in pieces (a whole Hubbard squash can weigh up to 20 pounds), this squash has a sweet and nutty flavor.

Pumpkin. Though more familiar in pie and jack-o'-lantern form, this rich, orange-rinded squash is delicious pureed, baked, or used to make soup.

Spaghetti. An oval-shaped squash with a pale yellow or beige rind. The stringy yellow flesh inside resembles spaghetti. When baked or steamed, the flesh makes a delicious, low-calorie substitute for pasta.

❖ Strawberries

The nutritional equivalent of a cup of broccoli, a cup of strawberries contains 141 percent of the recommended dietary allowance of vitamin C. Strawberries are also rich in dietary fiber and folic acid and contain fair amounts of potassium, iron, and riboflavin. In addition, ellagic acid, which may help keep healthy cells from becoming cancerous, is found in strawberries. And one cup of strawberries contains only 45 calories.

Cook's Note

Buy the freshest strawberries possible. Look for a deep red color, inside and out, and a fresh-looking, green cap. Strawberries do not ripen once they are picked, so select your berries carefully, checking for mold, bruises, or signs of too-long storage. Wash (and hull if necessary) strawberries just before you use them because they soak up liquid rapidly and can become waterlogged.

❖ Sunflower Seeds

Like pumpkin and corn, sunflowers are native to North America. The seeds were harvested by Native Americans long before Europeans arrived on these shores. Sunflower seeds are very high in nutrition: 1 ounce contains 6.5 grams of protein, 43 percent of the RDA for thiamin, 32 percent of the RDA for folate, and 29 percent of the RDA for magnesium (needed to help keep blood pressure regulated and build healthy nerves and muscles). Sunflower seeds also contain a good amount of iron, vitamin B_6, zinc, niacin, and potassium. Oil made from sunflower seeds is almost entirely monounsaturated or polyunsaturated, making it a healthy choice for cooking. In addition, 1 tablespoon of sunflower oil provides 61 percent of the RDA for vitamin E.

❖ Sweet Potatoes

What's the difference between a sweet potato and a yam? Sweet potatoes are native to the Americas. Columbus brought this light brown, orange-fleshed edible root back to Spain with him. Yams are native to Africa and Southeast Asia. Yams have a copper-colored skin and dark orange, syrupy-sweet flesh. Although the two roots are botanically different, the words have become basically interchangeable in common usage. To add to the confusion, many supermarkets call large sweet potatoes yams. True yams are hard to find. You'll probably have to seek them out at an ethnic market.

Nutritionally, sweet potatoes (which are not related to white potatoes) are an incredibly rich source of beta carotene. One medium baked sweet potato (about 4 ounces) provides 249 percent of your daily requirement for vitamin A. One sweet potato also has about half the RDA for vitamin C and valuable amounts of vitamin B_6, folic acid, potassium, riboflavin, magnesium, iron, and thiamine. That same single sweet potato also supplies 3.4 grams of dietary fiber and 27.7 grams of complex carbohydrates. The satisfying taste of a sweet potato makes it an excellent choice for dieters and diabetics.

Cook's Note

One pound of sweet potatoes averages out to roughly three medium-sized roots.

❖ Tea

A nice cup of tea can cheer you up—and also help prevent cancer, heart attacks, strokes, ulcers, osteoporosis, and even

tooth decay. Numerous studies have documented the value
of the various compounds found in green, oolong, and black
tea. (Herbal teas also have valuable uses, but there are far
too many to consider here.)

Tea is made from the leaves of *Camellia sinensis,* a
flowering evergreen plant native to parts of India and
China. Today, most tea is grown on plantations in India,
Sri Lanka, Indonesia, and China. Different types of tea are
the result of different ways of handling the fresh leaves.
Green tea, familiar from Asian restaurants, is made from
leaves that have been steamed, rolled, and then heated.
The final product is high in tannin, with a delicate per-
fume, a mild flavor, and a light color when brewed. Oolong tea is made by letting the fresh leaves wilt, rather
than steaming them. The leaves are then rolled and left to
ferment naturally for a time (for this reason, oolong tea is
also sometimes called semifermented tea). The leaves are
then heated to stop the fermentation process. Commercially, green tea is also sometimes called gunpowder or
hasten tea. Oolong tea is darker and more flavorful than
green tea; it has less tannin and less aroma. Black tea (the
familiar tea found in commercial tea bags) is made much
like oolong tea, but the fermentation process is allowed to
proceed longer. The flavor produced is strong and full.
Black tea is also sometimes called Pekoe or Orange Pekoe
tea. Flavorings are sometimes added to black tea; for example, Earl Grey is flavored with oil of bergamot, a citrus
fruit. All tea contains caffeine, but a cup of brewed tea has
far less caffeine than an equivalent cup of brewed coffee.
In general, green tea has less caffeine than black or oolong
tea.

Tea contains numerous substances that can contribute to
good health. Catechins, a chemical compound found in
tea, seem to help lower blood cholesterol levels and prevent atherosclerosis, or the buildup of dangerous plaque in
your arteries. Catechins may also help protect you against
cancer. A study in Japan suggests that people who drink a
lot of green tea are less likely to get stomach cancer.
Green tea has the most catechins and thus the most potent

anticancer effect; because catechins are reduced by the fermenting process, oolong and black teas have less. Tea also contains vitamin C, an antioxidant, and the minerals boron and manganese, both vital for strong bones and preventing osteoporosis. Drinking tea at the end of a meal could reduce your incidence of cavities, since tea contains antibiotic substances that can kill the germs that cause tooth decay.

Cook's Note

To brew a perfect pot of tea, bring fresh, cold water to a rapid boil. Pour about 1/4 cup of the hot water into the teapot and swirl the pot around to let the hot water warm the pot; discard the warming water. Place into the teapot 1 teaspoon of loose tea per cup, plus 1 teaspoon for the pot. Carefully pour the boiling water over the tea leaves. Place the lid on the teapot and let the tea steep for 3 to 5 minutes. Gently stir the tea once, then pour the tea into teacups, straining the liquid as you pour.

❖ Tofu (Bean Curd)

Tofu was once a strange and unusual food found only in Chinese restaurants and Oriental markets. Today, it is a familiar supermarket product, usually found in the produce section. Tofu is made by pouring coagulated soy milk into molds. The liquid drains off, leaving behind a soft, white cake with a very mild flavor. (Firmer tofu is pressed to remove more liquid.) Because it is made from soybeans, tofu offers many of the same health benefits as soybeans and is often the base for various soy food products. Tofu is often called "boneless meat" because of its high protein content—there are 12.8 grams of high-quality vegetable protein in a 3-ounce serving of firm tofu. An excellent dietary source of calcium, tofu is also a good source of iron, magnesium, folic acid, thiamine, and zinc as well. In addition, tofu is low in calories and virtually fat free.

Cook's Note

Fresh tofu can be stored in a container of water to cover in the refrigerator for up to a week. Change the water daily. Tofu can also be frozen for up to three months.

See also Soybeans.

❖ Tomatoes

Until well into this century, there were many people who believed tomatoes were poisonous, perhaps because tomatoes, like peppers, eggplants, and potatoes, are distantly related to the nightshade family of dangerous plants. Those who knew better prevailed, however, and today tomatoes are one of the largest vegetable crops in the world.

Tomatoes have a wide array of nutritional advantages. One fully ripe tomato has 39 percent of the RDA for vitamin C. Tomatoes can also give you about 6 percent of the RDA for iron, and the vitamin C makes it easier for your body to absorb. Dietary fiber and folic acid are present in tomatoes, as are vitamin A, potassium, and protein. The red color of tomatoes comes from lycopene, a carotenoid that has been shown to reduce the risk of certain cancers, including cancer of the bladder, cervix, lung, and particularly of the pancreas. The benefit of lycopenes is available from tomatoes in any form—even catsup. Although some people claim that eliminating all nightshade foods, including tomatoes, relieves their arthritis, there is very little scientific eivdence for the effectiveness of this approach.

❖ Triticale

A man-made contribution to the grain family, triticale (tri-ti-*kay*-lee) is a hybrid of wheat and rye that is available in many health food stores in the form of whole berries, flakes, and flour. In appearance, brown triticale berries look a great deal like wheat berries; the flavor is stronger than wheat, though, and the taste is sweet and nutty. With a higher protein content than either wheat or rye alone, a 1/2-cup serving of triticale contains 161 calories and 8.7 grams of dietary fiber. The same serving also offers 18 percent of the RDA for both folic acid and magnesium, 13 percent of the RDA for thiamin, 12 percent of the RDA for iron, and 11 percent of the RDA for zinc.

Like the rye from which it was bred, triticale is susceptible to ergot, a mold that can cause hallucinations, among other bizarre symptoms, so smell triticale carefully before using, and discard it if it has a musty, moldy smell.

Cook's Note
Triticale does contain some gluten, but for baked goods with superior texture, combine triticale flour with wheat flour. In its various whole grain forms, triticale usually requires presoaking and long cooking.

❖ Turnip Greens

Often cut off and thrown away, turnip greens contain amazing amounts of many vitamins and minerals, considerably more than the turnip root itself. An exceptional source of dietary fiber (1.4 grams per 1/2-cup serving), turnip greens are chock-full of beta carotene (a 1/2-cup serving of cooked turnip greens contains more than 75 percent of the RDA for vitamin A), and a generous dose of vitamin C. Turnip greens also offer large amounts of calcium.

Cook's Note
Turnip greens can be prepared and used as you would fresh spinach. And like spinach, turnip greens may be gritty and should be washed thoroughly before using.

❖ Walnuts

Nuts in general are good for you, and walnuts are no exception. This popular nut is available in two varieties: black and English walnuts. Black walnuts are native to North America. They have very hard shells that are difficult to crack; the nut itself has a strong flavor. For this reason, black walnuts are not widely available. The English walnut, known also as the Persian or California walnut, is the most common walnut sold today. Over half of the English walnuts sold commercially are grown in the United States, primarily in California. English walnuts are easy to shell and mild in taste.

Walnuts provide fiber and some vitamins and minerals, but their chief nutritional benefit is their high oil content. Walnuts are the best vegetable source of omega-3 fatty acids, the same monounsaturated fat in fish oil. Omega-3 fatty acids can help reduce your blood cholesterol levels, protect you against heart disease, and fight cancer. In addition, walnuts are high in ellagic acid, another antioxidant substance that can help prevent atherosclerosis and coronary artery disease. Walnuts are also high in calories. Fortunately, you can get the benefits of walnuts by eating just three or four a day.

See also Nuts.

❖ Water

Your body consists of about 70 percent water, so the importance of having enough water in the diet cannot be expressed too often or stressed too much. You can live without food for weeks, but you would die in just a few days without water. You need water to transport nutrients to all the cells in the body and remove wastes quickly. Today, most doctors and nutritionists recommend drinking six to eight 8-ounce glasses of water a day—or even more in very hot weather or if you are very active. It's almost impossible to drink too much water—whatever your body can't use is disposed of efficiently through the kidneys. (If you have kidney disease, heart failure, or some other serious condition, discuss how much water to drink with your doctor.)

Drinking a lot of water is also a good way to prevent kidney stones, relieve the symptoms of bladder infections, replenish fluids lost to diarrhea, vomiting, or athletic activity, prevent constipation, and maintain normal body temperature and blood pressure.

In almost all cases, there's nothing wrong with plain tap water straight from the sink. Your local water supply is generally filtered and treated to remove impurities and microorganisms. In many communities, small amounts of fluoride are added to the water to help prevent tooth decay. It is possible, however, that your tap water can pick up impurities such as lead and copper from corroded pipes in your household plumbing. Due to local water treatment procedures, tap water can sometimes have a faintly unpleasant taste or odor. Simple filtration systems usually solve this problem.

If you live in an area where the water is noticeably hard (in other words, has a high mineral content), you may wish to drink bottled water to avoid the mineral taste. Many people prefer bottled water in general, feeling that it is purer and tastes and smells better than tap water. Mineral water, which by definition contains minerals such as calcium and magnesium, is a popular choice. Another type of bottled water is spring water. This water is taken from natural water sources that have varying degrees of mineral content. Both mineral and spring waters are usually filtered to remove impurities and microorganisms; some mineral and spring waters are naturally carbonated, while others are still. One word of warning: Children who drink nothing but bottled water may not be getting enough fluoride to prevent tooth decay. Discuss the importance of fluoride for children with your dentist.

❖ Watermelon

Believe it or not, watermelon is actually a vegetable. In fact, watermelon is kin to the cucumber. Native to Africa, watermelons are now grown worldwide. This ever-popular melon has a thick, dark green or green and white striped rind and vivid pink flesh with numerous black seeds. Depending on the variety, watermelons can range in size from small, round melons weighing 4 to 10 pounds to huge, oblong 45-pounders. Seedless or yellow-fleshed varieties are now available.

Watermelons get their lovely pink color from lycopene, a carotenoid that has been shown to reduce the risk of certain cancers, particularly of the pancreas. Watermelon is an excellent source of dietary fiber and has a surprisingly large amount of vitamin C—26 percent of the RDA in a 1-cup serving. It also has surprisingly few calories for a fruit that tastes so sweet. There's just 51 calories in a serving.

See also Melons.

❖ Wheat Bran

A kernel or berry of wheat is the seed of the wheat plant. It consists of the bran (the outer hull of the kernel), the endosperm (the interior of the kernel), and the germ (the sprouting section at the base of the endosperm).

Wheat kernels are ground to make flour. If the bran is left on the kernel before grinding, the result is whole wheat flour. If the bran is removed, the result is white flour.

Wheat bran (also sometimes called miller's bran) is sold separately in health food stores. It can vary in color from tan to dark red brown. Depending on the method of milling, the consistency ranges from powdery to flaky. Its primary use is as a supplement to provide dietary fiber, but wheat bran is also a good source of B vitamins and copper. There's some evidence to suggest that eating wheat bran can reduce a woman's risk of breast cancer by lowering the levels of estrogen in the blood. Wheat bran also contains phytate, a substance that has been shown to prevent colon cancer in animals—and possibly in humans as well.

❖ Wheat Germ

The germ in wheat germ isn't a bacteria. Rather, it is the tiny portion of a wheat kernel that sprouts when the seed is planted. Because it is high in oil, the germ is often removed from the kernel when milling wheat for flour; otherwise, the flour would become rancid if not used quickly. Wheat germ is slightly crunchy and has a delicious, slightly nutty flavor that is packed with nutrition. A quarter cup of wheat germ has 8.3 grams of high-quality protein, 3.7 grams of insoluble dietary fiber, and is an excellent source of vitamin E, folic acid, riboflavin, niacin, zinc, thiamine, iron, magnesium, and potassium.

As health foods go, wheat germ is unusually palatable. It can be added to casseroles, baked goods, and pancakes, or sprinkled on oatmeal, yogurt, fruit, or anything else.

Cook's Note

The high fat content in wheat germ can cause it to spoil quickly. Store it in a sealed container in the refrigerator for up to six months.

❖ Wild Rice

Not a rice at all, wild rice is the seed of a kind of wild grass that grows primarily in the Great Lakes region of North America. Purple black or dark brown in color, wild rice is chewy in texture and pleasantly nutty in taste. A 1/2-cup serving contains 83 calories, very little fat, and 3.3 grams of protein. Wild rice also offers a rich array of vitamins and minerals, including folic acid, magnesium, zinc, niacin, and vitamin B_6.

Cook's Note

Soak wild rice before using and discard any debris floating on the surface. Wild rice is a bit expensive (mostly due to harvesting costs). To stretch it further, make it into a pilaf with white or brown rice.

❖ Wine

Wine has been honored for its medicinal properties since the days of ancient Greece. Recent research suggests that wine, particularly red wine, could help lower your risk of coronary artery disease. Moderate consumption of wine—no more than two glasses a day—may help raise the level of good cholesterol in the blood. In fact, numerous studies have documented that moderate wine drinkers tend to have a lower incidence of heart disease and lower blood pressure. In addition, red wine contains a substance called resveratrol that can help prevent dangerous blood clots that could lead to a stroke or heart attack. (Resveratrol comes from the skins of grapes, so it is not found in white wine.) The key, of course, is the word *moderate*. If you don't drink at all or drink only occasionally, it's probably not worth starting to get the benefits of red wine. If you have any chronic health problem such as diabetes or angina, or if you regularly take medication (prescription or nonprescription) for any condition, discuss drinking red wine or any alcohol with your doctor.

Alcohol in general, and red wine in particular, can trigger migraine headaches for some people. If you're trying to conceive, are pregnant or think you might be, or if you are breast-feeding, avoid all alcohol, including wine.

❖ Yams
See Sweet Potatoes.

❖ Yogurt

If you are one of the millions of women who suffer from recurrent vaginal yeast infections, eating yogurt could help. Yogurt containing active cultures may significantly reduce the occurrence and severity of these highly uncomfortable infections. *Lactobacillus acidophilus,* the microorganism that turns milk into yogurt, seems to raise your level of gamma interferon, which helps your immune system to fight disease. This may help fight vaginitis, prevent some colds, and lower the risk of other infections. The infection-fighting power of yogurt is found only in the live-culture kind. Read the labels on the yogurt in the supermarket dairy case carefully. If you can't find live-culture yogurt there, try your health food store.

Any kind of yogurt is a good source of dietary calcium, particularly for people who are lactose intolerant and can't drink milk. One cup of low-fat yogurt gives you about half the recommended dietary allowance.

An expert on nutrition, **Dr. David Kessler** has had an active New York practice, specializing in family medicine, for over twenty years. Dr. Kessler received his M.D. from Albany Medical College. In addition, he was recently named a diplomate of the National Board of Examiners, and is a diplomate of the American Board of Family Practice.

Sheila Buff is a professional medical writer and the author of over twenty books to date including *All About Non-prescription Drugs and Vitamins*. In addition, she is the Managing Director of Ibid. Editorial Services.

From the editors of
PREVENTION
The #1 Health Magazine